T0114568

THE BASICS OF
REIKI

THE BASICS OF
REIKI

*A step-by-step guide
to healing with Reiki*

PENELOPE QUEST

JEREMY P. TARCHER / PENGUIN
a member of Penguin Group (USA) Inc.
New York

JEREMY P. TARCHER/PENGUIN
Published by the Penguin Group
Penguin Group (USA) Inc., 375 Hudson Street, New York, New York 10014, USA ·
Penguin Group (Canada), 90 Eglinton Avenue East, Suite 700, Toronto, Ontario M4P 2Y3, Canada
(a division of Pearson Penguin Canada Inc.) · Penguin Books Ltd, 80 Strand, London WC2R 0RL,
England · Penguin Ireland, 25 St Stephen's Green, Dublin 2, Ireland (a division of Penguin Books Ltd) ·
Penguin Group (Australia), 707 Collins Street, Melbourne, Victoria 3008, Australia (a division of
Pearson Australia Group Pty Ltd) · Penguin Books India Pvt Ltd, 11 Community Centre, Panchsheel Park,
New Delhi–110 017, India · Penguin Group (NZ), 67 Apollo Drive, Rosedale, Auckland 0632,
New Zealand (a division of Pearson New Zealand Ltd) · Penguin Books (South Africa), Rosebank Office Park,
181 Jan Smuts Avenue, Parktown North 2193, South Africa · Penguin China, B7 Jiaming Center,
27 East Third Ring Road North, Chaoyang District, Beijing 100020, China

Penguin Books Ltd, Registered Offices: 80 Strand, London WC2R 0RL, England

First published in Great Britain in 2007 by Piatkus Books Ltd
Copyright © 2007 by Penelope Quest

ISBN 978-0-399-16220-6

Neither the publisher nor the author is engaged in rendering professional advice or services to the
individual reader. The ideas, procedures, and suggestions contained in this book are not intended as a
substitute for consulting with your physician. All matters regarding your health require medical supervision.
Neither the author nor the publisher shall be liable or responsible for any loss or damage allegedly arising from any
information or suggestion in this book.

While the author has made every effort to provide accurate telephone numbers, Internet addresses,
and other contact information at the time of publication, neither the publisher nor the author assumes
any responsibility for errors, or for changes that occur after publication. Further, the publisher does not have any control
over and does not assume any rsponsibility for author or third-party websites or their content.

This book is dedicated to Mikao Usui, and to his students, without whom the world would not have received the wonderful gift of Reiki.

CONTENTS

ACKNOWLEDGMENTS

I would like to express my heartfelt gratitude to the many people who have helped, directly or indirectly, with this book, especially to my Reiki teachers, Kristin Bonney, William Lee Rand, Andy Bowling, Richard Rivard and Robert Jefford, and to my many Reiki students, for the love and learning they have brought me. I would also like to thank the many Reiki friends I have made all over the world for their ideas and inspiration, and in particular the members of the UK Reiki Federation (UKRF) and the Reiki Regulation Working Group (RRWG). Many thanks also to the Piatkus editing and production staff, especially Gill, Helen, Allie, Krystyna and Briony, and to Rodney for his excellent illustrations.

INTRODUCTION

Nowadays it is not unusual to see articles about Reiki in newspapers and magazines, or to hear about it on the radio or in TV programs, but back in 1990, when I first encountered it, it was pretty remarkable. I have always been interested in esoteric and alternative subjects, and began my search for personal and spiritual development in the mid-1970s, studying anything and everything from astrology, cartomancy and graphology to numerology, palmistry and even social psychology. One evening in 1990 I attended a talk on personal growth techniques, and I was really impressed by the speaker, Kristin Bonney, mainly because she seemed so calm and tranquil—and tranquility was completely absent from my own life at the time. I was then living a ridiculously frenetic lifestyle as a single parent, working long hours as a college lecturer, and studying in what I laughingly called my "spare" time for an Open University degree.

While chatting with someone during the coffee break I was told that Kristin practiced and taught a hands-on healing technique called Reiki, which I had never heard of, so a few months later I went along to one of her introductory talks on the subject, and I found it fascinating. I had my first experience of Reiki flowing through me as I sat on the floor in front of a Reiki practitioner, and while Kristin talked the practitioner simply placed his hands on my shoulders. Almost immediately I could feel this wonderful, flowing softness, gentleness, warmth and tingling flooding through my body. I could feel emotions welling up inside me, even though I felt quite relaxed and peaceful, and I could sense a soothing progress down my body, into my legs, and right into my feet and toes. It was the most astonishing sensation, and after only fifteen minutes I felt fantastic. I decided right there and then that Reiki was something I really wanted in my life.

It took a while for me to find some free time, but in 1991 I attended a weekend Reiki First Degree course, and I will admit I went along in some trepidation, not sure what to expect. I had always assumed that "healers" were special people, born with unique gifts, so surely an ordinary person like myself couldn't become a healer, and certainly not in just a couple of days? I also thought that even if it could work for some of the students attending that course, it probably wouldn't work for me. Of course, on both counts I was proved wrong—and now, having taught Reiki myself for many years, I realize that most students feel like that when they come along to their first Reiki course.

Kristin reassured me that we *all* have the potential to be healers, and even by the end of the first day I could feel a lovely warm energy flowing from my hands when I tried to use Reiki on myself. By the end of the second day I had received my first Reiki treatment, and had successfully carried out one on another student. I went out of that class a Reiki evangelist! I thought it was the most wonderful thing in the world, and couldn't wait to try it out on my family, friends, cats—and anything or anyone else that would stand still long enough!

Soon I started a part-time Reiki practice, fitting it into my busy life with surprising ease, and a year later I felt it was time to take the Reiki Second Degree course, which was even more amazing. It was as though the whole world around me had changed—colors were brighter, sounds were sharper, smells and tastes were more intense—as if a veil had been lifted and I was seeing the world for the first time. My awareness was incredibly enhanced, and I felt a tremendous connection to everything around me, from people, animals and plants, to rocks and water. It felt truly magical, and for me it seemed as though I had taken an enormous leap forward spiritually. Over the weeks and months that followed, as I practiced the new skills I had been taught, I discovered that my intuition and psychic abilities were growing rapidly, so that I became fully clairvoyant, clairaudient and clairsentient. I even began to "see" inside my clients' bodies, so that I could tell what was wrong with them—although, as you can imagine, the first few times that happened was a shock, and a bit frightening. I'd thought X-ray vision was an invention of comic-book heroes like Superman! However, if you find that prospect a bit alarming, I can say that this doesn't happen to everyone who does Reiki; I think Reiki just boosts your potential in whatever gifts are inherent within you.

Over the next couple of years I continued to give Reiki treatments at home, and began to give talks about it to interested groups. In August 1994 I became a Reiki Master, the term applied to those who have done Reiki Third

Degree who then become teachers of this healing art. That was a profound and moving spiritual experience for me, beyond anything I had previously known, and I soon realized that I had only just taken my first few steps on a very special spiritual path *toward* the mastery of Reiki, because being a Reiki Master is a lifelong commitment to personal growth and spiritual development, as well as to a deep and powerful understanding of healing on all levels—physical, emotional, psychological and spiritual. At the end of 1995 I took the plunge and gave up my job in education management to become a Reiki Master full time, teaching and writing about Reiki and other mind/body healing techniques, which I believe is my true vocation.

Reiki has transformed my life, and I am happier now than I have ever been. I believe I am living the life I was meant to live, following the spiritual path I was meant to follow. Reiki is there in my hands whenever I need it, and it has led me to many interesting experiences and taught me so much, and through it I have met hundreds of lovely people. It has been a pleasure and a privilege to help so many to experience the joy and wonder of those first moments when the Reiki flows through their hands, and to see some of them progress to become Reiki Masters themselves, handing on their knowledge and experience to even more Reiki students.

My aim in this book is to provide a comprehensive and accessible introduction to the subject of Reiki—where it came from, how it works, what it is like to receive a treatment, how easy it is to learn and what you can do with it. I believe that when the time is right, and you have reached a particular stage in your own personal path of spiritual development, Reiki begins to turn up in your life—Reiki finds you, rather than you finding Reiki. Maybe that's why this book has turned up for you now. I hope you find it interesting and informative. Perhaps it will inspire you to book an appointment for a Reiki treatment, or even to take your first Reiki course. In whatever way is right for you, I wish you joy on your journey with Reiki.

PENELOPE QUEST

THE BASICS OF
REIKI

part one

WHAT IS REIKI?

chapter one

THE ORIGINS OF REIKI
AS A HEALING SYSTEM

The Japanese word Reiki (pronounced "RAY-KEE") means "spiritual energy," or "universal life-force energy," and in Japan the word is used to describe any healing method that utilizes spiritual energy—i.e., forms of spiritual healing. However, the word Reiki in the West normally refers to a particular healing energy practice discovered in the early part of the twentieth century by a Japanese scholar, Dr. Mikao Usui (1865–1926). After many years of research he found a way of drawing into himself and others a form of spiritual energy for healing and spiritual development, which became known as Usui Reiki Ryoho, meaning the Usui Spiritual Energy Healing Method. (This is sometimes known as Usui Shiki Ryoho, which is usually translated as the Usui System of Natural Healing.)

In the Japanese alphabet, or kanji, Reiki is really composed of two words—Rei and Ki, and it is represented calligraphically like this:

靈　靈
氣　気

On the left is the Reiki kanji as it would have been written in Dr. Usui's time, and on the right is a more modern version. In both cases, the top pictogram represents "Rei," and the bottom one represents "Ki." The Japanese language is very complex, so each word/kanji can have many possible meanings.

REI	Universal, boundless, transcendental, spirit, soul, divine, sacred, essence, mysterious power, God's wisdom, higher power, supernatural knowledge, spiritual consciousness
KI	Spiritual energy, life-force energy, cosmic energy (also represented in other languages as Chi, Qi, Prana, Mana, Light, Holy Ghost or Holy Spirit)

As you can see, there are a number of ways of interpreting the word Reiki, but one way to summarize this is:

- "**Rei**" can be understood as the Higher Intelligence that guides the creation and functioning of the universe; the wisdom that comes from God (or the Source, the Creator, the Universe, the All-That-Is), which is all knowing, and which understands the need for, and cause of, all problems and difficulties and how to heal them.
- "**Ki**" is the life-force energy that flows through every living thing—plants, animals and people—and that is present in some form in everything around us, even rocks and inanimate objects.

When these words are put together, therefore, the meaning of Reiki is simplified as "spiritual energy," "soul energy" or "universal life-force energy"—a form of energy that is guided by a subtle wisdom to heal all aspects of the person—body, mind and spirit.

SO WHAT IS REIKI?

The way in which Reiki is seen in the West today is primarily as a form of complementary therapy—a safe, gentle, nonintrusive hands-on healing technique that uses spiritual energy to treat physical ailments without the need for massage or manipulation. But it is much more than a physical therapy. It is a holistic system for balancing, healing and harmonizing the mind, emotions and spirit, as well as the physical body, promoting a sense of well-being.

So Reiki is healing energy, but healing in its most all-encompassing sense. Healing the physical, mental, emotional and spiritual aspects enables a person to become whole, or "holy" in what was probably the original sense of the word. Also, unlike other complementary or alternative therapies, the practice of Reiki is a spiritual discipline that includes meditation, energy-cleansing techniques and spiritual principles for living, and practitioners are encouraged to use Reiki on themselves daily, not only for self-healing, but also to increase self-awareness, personal growth and spiritual development.

Reiki is therefore a connection to the essence of life itself, and as such is a gift of immeasurable proportions. It is guided by a higher wisdom and always works for the highest good of the person receiving it, so it can do no harm.

THE ORIGINS OF REIKI

We may never know the exact origins of Reiki as a healing system, but it probably dates back at least 2,500 years, as we know that the Buddha used something similar, and it is likely to be even older than that. However, the healing system we use today in the West was developed initially by Dr. Mikao Usui in Japan, and further developed by one of his students, Dr. Chujiro Hayashi, who passed his teachings on to a Hawaiian woman of Japanese parentage, Mrs. Hawayo Takata.

THE REIKI STORY

Since the early 1990s there have been various versions of the Reiki history, the earlier accounts relying on the knowledge of Mrs. Takata, the person who originally brought Reiki to the West in the late 1930s, and later reports that have been based on research carried out in Japan.

Mrs. Takata taught Reiki as an oral system, so the story was handed down from teacher to student, and in her version the founder of the system, Dr. Mikao Usui, was a Christian priest who became fascinated by the stories of Jesus healing people, so he spent many years studying, learning languages and traveling out of Japan to other countries, including the U.S.A., in order to find out the secret of healing. He failed to find the information he was seeking in Christian texts, but when he studied the Sanskrit Sutras and Japanese Lotus Sutras (spiritual texts) he found what he was looking for, yet despite this he could not activate his own ability to heal. However, at a Zen Buddhist monastery he was advised to go on retreat to meditate in order to find the answer, and this he did.

At the end of a 21-day fasting retreat at Mount Kurama, he was apparently struck by a great light, and saw the sacred symbols he had discovered during his research; he acquired a deep understanding of these symbols, received a spiritual empowerment and achieved enlightenment. When the retreat was over, despite his weakness after 21 days of fasting, he rushed down the mountain in great excitement, but he injured his foot in his haste, and when he bent down to hold his sore toe, he found that the bleeding stopped, the pain went away and he was healed. When he reached the bottom of the mountain he sought out a food seller. His meal was brought to him by a young girl, and he noticed that she had a swollen, tear-smeared face. She told him she had a very bad toothache, but her father could not afford to send her for treatment. Remembering his success at healing his foot, he asked if he could place his hands on her face to see if it would help—very quickly, the swelling and pain were gone. Later, on reaching the monastery to discuss his revelations, he was told that the Abbot had taken to his bed with severe arthritis, and he was again able to help by placing his hands on the Abbot's painful joints. Thus he had proof that he had finally discovered the healing power for which he had been searching.

Mrs. Takata told her students that Usui spent many years healing people in Japan before eventually passing on his teachings to Dr. Chujiro Hayashi (1879–1940), a commander in the Japanese Navy. After Usui's death Hayashi was said to have opened a Reiki clinic, which was where Hawayo Takata (1900-1980), a young woman from Hawaii who was visiting relatives in Japan, came to be healed of a serious illness. She was so impressed with the success of her treatment that she begged to be able to learn Reiki. Hayashi eventually agreed to teach her, and she lived with his family and worked without pay in his clinic in exchange for the privilege of being able to learn the first and second levels of this healing system. In due course she went back to Hawaii and opened the first Reiki clinic in the West. In 1938 Hayashi and his family visited her, and he passed on the final level of the Reiki teachings so that she would be able to teach this healing art to others. Mrs. Takata believed that all of Hayashi's Reiki students in Japan were killed during the Second World War, and that she was therefore the only Reiki teacher left alive.

Mrs. Takata continued to teach Reiki and run her clinic

in Hawaii, but also began to travel extensively throughout the U.S.A. and Canada, treating people with Reiki and training them how to use it for themselves. She held classes in the first two levels of Reiki training, which she called First Degree and Second Degree, but it was the 1970s before she began to pass on the final level of teachings, the Third Degree, which she called Reiki Master (a rough translation of "sensei," meaning respected teacher in Japanese), so that others would be able to continue to spread Reiki when she had gone. By the time of her death in December 1980, after 42 years of teaching Reiki, she had trained 22 Masters, and it is through them that Reiki has spread so widely throughout the Western world.

NEW INFORMATION ABOUT REIKI

In the late 1990s new information began to come to the West from Japan, which showed that Usui had been a Buddhist scholar, not a Christian priest, and that he had passed his complete teachings on to about 20 people, including five Buddhist nuns, so Chujiro Hayashi had not been his only Master-level student. It was discovered that not all the Reiki Masters in Japan had, after all, been killed during the Second World War, and it became apparent that Reiki had continued to be taught there after Mikao Usui's death. Indeed, an organization had existed from Usui's time that was dedicated to preserving his original teachings—the Usui Reiki Ryoho Gakkai—which held his original teaching manuals, the *Hikkei*. This fuller and more accurate picture of Reiki's discovery and development came particularly from two men—Frank Arjava Petter, a German Reiki Master then living and working in Japan with his Japanese wife, Chetna Kobayashi, and Hiroshi Doi, a Japanese Reiki Master who has trained in both Japanese and Western Reiki traditions. Others who have contributed to our current knowledge of Japanese Reiki include Dave King, Melissa Riggall, Robert Jefford, Andy Bowling and Rick Rivard, all of whom have spent time researching Reiki history in Japan.

THE BACKGROUND TO THE DISCOVERY OF REIKI

We now know that Usui was born in Japan on August 15, 1865, and that he began his study of Buddhism at the age of four, when he was sent to a monastery school run by the Tendai Buddhist sect. He studied martial arts from the age of 12, reaching the highest levels of Menkyo Kaiden by his midtwenties and of other ancient Japanese systems as he got older, including Ki-kou, the Japanese form of a martial art and energy-balancing system similar to the better known Chi Kung from China. He additionally learned meditation and healing, and studied other forms of Buddhism. He also worked in many different jobs, and had a wife and children, so he was not a cloistered monk.

During Usui's lifetime the political climate in Japan changed radically, especially during the reign of Emperor Mutsuhito, who initiated the more receptive Meiji Restoration Period (1868–1912). Japan's previously closed borders were opened for the first time in many centuries, allowing Japanese people, and especially scholars, to explore Western languages, sciences and industrial methods.

Usui's memorial, in the graveyard of the Saihoji temple in Tokyo, confirms that he traveled widely, visiting China, Europe and the U.S.A., acquiring knowledge of medicine, history, psychology and world religions. It also confirms that he had a mystical enlightenment experience on Mount Kurama, near Kyoto, and that he spent the few years before his death at the age of 60 (March 9, 1926) practicing and teaching his healing system, and passing on his knowledge to others so that the teachings could continue. His memorial states:

If Reiki can be spread throughout the world it will touch the human heart and the morals of society. It will be helpful for many people, not only healing disease, but the earth as a whole.

chapter two

THE GROWTH OF REIKI
IN THE WEST

As I indicated in Chapter 1, we owe a great debt of gratitude to Mrs. Hawayo Takata, because without her it is possible that none of us in the West would have heard of Reiki, and certainly we would not be able to practice it or teach it. She established a system of teaching Reiki that survives to this day, through the lineage of some of the 22 Masters she taught, although since the early 1990s there have been a number of changes made, which are outlined later in this chapter.

It seems that Mrs. Takata adapted the teaching of Reiki to suit Western students, for example teaching First Degree or Second Degree as workshops held over just a few days, to fit in with most Western working lives, rather than expecting students to work in her clinic for months in order to learn, as she had done in Hayashi's clinic in Japan. Her priority seems to have been not only to treat individuals with Reiki, but also to train them and their family in Reiki so that they could continue the treatments regularly. She used a series of 12 basic hand positions for both self-treatment and treatment of others, which she called the "Foundation Treatment," and she encouraged her Reiki students to work on themselves with Reiki every day. Also, she advised that each hand position should last five minutes, and recommended that students carry out four or more treatments on each client for maximum benefit. In addition, realizing that in the West her students related money to importance, and wanting people to value the incredible gift of Reiki, she charged high course fees—$150 for Reiki 1, $500 for Reiki 2, and $10,000 for Reiki 3 (Reiki Master). To put this into context, in the early 1970s when Takata began to teach Reiki Masters, $10,000 would buy a house in the U.S.A., so she was expecting a tremendous commitment from the students who chose to become Reiki Masters—she expected them to dedicate their lives to Reiki, as she had done.

THE FORMATION OF THE REIKI ALLIANCE

After Hawayo Takata's death, a group of the Masters she had taught met in Hawaii in 1982 to discuss how Reiki should progress, and who should become the next leader, the title they used being "Grand Master." This may have been how Takata had described herself, since she had believed she was the only Reiki Master in the West for so many years. It appears there were two "favorites" for the post—Phyllis Lei Furumoto, Mrs. Takata's granddaughter, and Barbara Weber Ray. Phyllis agreed to follow in her grandmother's footsteps and was therefore elected by the majority of the Masters. Soon afterward Dr. Barbara Weber Ray broke away to found her own system of

Reiki, called the Radiance Technique, which she later renamed Real Reiki.

That historic first meeting in 1982 allowed Western Reiki Masters to share their experiences for the first time, and they discovered differences in the way they had been taught, perhaps because Mrs. Takata had taught the system as an oral tradition, not even allowing her student Masters to take notes. They therefore took some decisions that have had a major influence on the development of Reiki in the West. They standardized the system, agreeing on the nine elements of Reiki teaching, and at a further meeting in British Columbia in 1983 the Reiki Masters formed the Reiki Alliance, an organization of Reiki Masters who recognized Phyllis Lei Furumoto as the Grand Master, and whose purpose was to support one another as teachers of the Usui system of Reiki. Some Masters, especially those who belong to the Reiki Alliance, keep to these exact traditions, although as I explain later, the majority of Masters today teach the system differently.

The Nine Elements of Teaching the Usui System of Reiki Healing

An oral tradition The teaching of Reiki requires that the Reiki Master and student should be physically present together for the initiations, the history and the personal guidance through the forms of self-treatment and treatment of others.

Spiritual lineage	The spiritual lineage is seen as the embodiment of the essence of the Usui system, and is carried from Dr. Usui through Hayashi and Takata to the 22 Masters she taught, and from them through to other Masters.
History	The story of the rediscovery of Reiki by Dr. Usui is told in classes as part of the oral tradition.
Precepts for daily living	The five spiritual principles of Reiki as taught by Takata were: 1. Just for today, do not anger; 2. Just for today, do not worry; 3. Honor your parents, teachers and elders; 4. Do your work honestly; 5. Show gratitude to every living thing. (Some variations exist between individual Masters.)
Form of classes	Three Degrees or levels make up the Usui system. There are specific requirements for what must be taught at each level, and a minimum amount of time is required for this teaching (12 hours each for Reiki 1 and 2, unlimited up to one year or more for Reiki 3), as well as a recommended time span between classes—three months between Reiki 1 and Reiki 2, and three years experience of Reiki before undertaking Reiki 3 (Master level).
Money (exchange)	The Reiki Alliance still recommends the fees originally set by Hawayo Takata: $150 for Reiki 1, $500 for Reiki 2 and $10,000 for Reiki Master.

Initiation	The initiation or attunement process is a sacred ritual which, when performed by a Master with a student, results in the student's capacity to channel Reiki. There are four initiations for Reiki 1, one for Reiki 2 and one for Reiki Master.
Symbols	There are four Reiki symbols which act as energetic keys, when used in conjunction with Reiki, and these are intended to be kept sacred, and are only taught to students of Second Degree (three symbols) and Master level (one symbol).
Treatment	Self-treatment is the first priority, before the treatment of others. There are specific forms of 12 hand positions for each treatment— four on the head, four on the front of the body and four on the back of the body. (There are other variations of this, with some of Takata's Masters teaching between 16 and 20 hand placements, such as extra positions on the head, and including hand placements on the legs and feet.)

The Expansion of the System

Until 1988, only Phyllis Lei Furumoto, as Grand Master, was entitled to train other Masters, but in a gathering at Friedricksburg that year she announced that any suitably experienced Master could teach other Masters. This significant decision is what opened up Reiki in the West to the inevitable changes that result from expansion, as by the early 1990s the number of Masters and practitioners had grown extensively all over the world. A growing number of Masters moved away from the system agreed by the Reiki Alliance to work independently, changing the way they taught Reiki, especially the way they taught the Master level. Instead of an apprenticeship system, where one or two trainee Masters would work alongside an established Master for a year or more, the Reiki Third Degree began to be taught in large groups in courses lasting just a few days.

This resulted in a massive expansion in the number of Masters, with a consequent growth in the number of people learning First and Second Degree Reiki, so that Reiki rapidly spread all over the world. Since the late 1990s the Reiki Alliance, along with Phyllis Lei Furumoto and another of Takata's Masters, Paul Mitchell, have been actively encouraging Masters and practitioners to come into alignment with their approved system, but with little success. Reiki is now so widespread, and there are so many different versions of Usui's original healing system being taught in the West, that it is probably an impossible task to try to standardize Reiki.

Changes in the System

Since the early 1990s many things have changed in the way Reiki is taught by Reiki Masters who do not belong to the Reiki Alliance. For example, the cost of Reiki courses varies enormously: very few Masters now adhere to the prices set by Mrs. Takata, so it is possible to learn Reiki very inexpensively, for a moderate sum or for a lot of money. The choice is yours, although clearly different things may be offered and this may have an impact on what a potential Reiki student decides to pay. Also, the system is no longer regarded as a purely oral tradition. Most Masters now give out manuals or handouts to their students. Many—perhaps most—modern Reiki Masters do not observe the time span requirements between levels. Some teach Reiki 1 on a Saturday and Reiki 2 immediately afterward on the Sunday, with perhaps Reiki 3 a few weeks later, and a few even teach all three levels in a week, or even in a weekend. Quite a lot of Masters now just offer attunements (the method of passing on the ability to channel the Reiki energy) at each of the levels, without any tuition in how to use Reiki for self-treatment or the treatment of others. I explain more about the ways in which Reiki can be taught in Chapter 7.

chapter three

THE TRADITIONS IN JAPAN

It is a facet of Japanese culture that knowledge or important information is normally kept secret (or sacred, as the words are synonymous in the Japanese language) within family groups, so initially Usui used Reiki only on himself and his family, and it is reported that Reiki cured his wife of a serious illness at that time. However, he eventually realized how important his discovery was, and began to teach people how to access this healing energy, making Shoden (the first level of Reiki training) "freely available to all of the people"—a direct quote from one of his teaching manuals, the *Usui Reiki Hikkei*.

It is believed that Usui taught Reiki at three levels:

1. Shoden (meaning "the entrance").
2. Okuden (meaning "the deep inside").
3. Shinpiden (meaning "the mystery/secret teachings").

This would certainly equate with the three levels that are currently taught in the West—i.e., First Degree, Second Degree and Third Degree/Reiki Master. Usui is thought to have taught the first level of Reiki to about 2,000 people, although it is understood that he called it Teate, meaning "healing hands," or "palm healing," rather than Reiki. Of these 2,000, Usui apparently taught between 30 and 50 people the second level, but only about 20 acquired the third level, and it is even possible that some of these may not have completed the full training in this final step. This may have been because some of them, such as Chujiro Hayashi, were Christians and therefore it might have been viewed as inappropriate that they be taught some of the more sacred Buddhist teachings. However, it may also have been because, in the tradition of many spiritual masters before him, Mikao Usui may only have taught Reiki for a few years, from 1922 to 1926.

In April 1922 Dr. Usui is believed to have opened his first clinic, in Harajuku, Tokyo, where he practiced and taught Reiki. His healing skills must have been extraordinary, as he was renowned all over Japan, and admired as "the pioneer of restarting Hands-on Healing from past generations," which is another quote from his memorial.

However, the emphasis of Usui's teaching was concerned with spiritual practice to bring about a spiritual awakening, rather than with purely physical healing. Indeed, there was nothing unique in his Teate, or "palm healing" method, as it was similar to other healing methods in Japan at that time. His true uniqueness comes from his spiritual teachings. Suzuki-san, one of Usui's original Shinpiden students who was 106 in 2005, when one of my Reiki Masters met her, was drawn to him by these teachings, and not by the healing method, which she learned only as a side issue. Her concern was that the "spiritual teachings" of Mikao Usui should be preserved—

that is, the spiritual path undertaken by Usui which resulted in the birth of Reiki. Here is a quote from Suzuki-san:

> These are "Special Teachings," not Secret.
> They need to be taught from person to person.
> They cannot be taught any other way.
> The teachings need to be tailored to each individual.
> Each individual's experience is different.

What this means is that in Japan students do not receive teachings until they are ready. People often speak about the spiritual aspect of Reiki or Usui's teachings, but in the West we have turned things around. To most Western people, Reiki is a healing system with some interesting spiritual aspects, whereas Usui's emphasis was really on a spiritual practice with healing as an interesting side effect!

Usui never claimed to be a Shihan (Master), referring to his teachings as the "method to achieve personal perfection." He taught that by mastering the mysteries of the self we learn to affect the mysteries of life, so his teachings are about "personal mastery"—the healing of the Self.

> You are everything. If you are healing yourself you heal everything.
>
> (A quote attributed to Usui)

Usui passed on a series of spiritual and energy disciplines that encapsulated his wisdom gained over nearly 50 years of spiritual practice, including that extraordinary enlightenment experience on Mount Kurama, and while the teachings require specific guidance from experienced teachers, they were not regarded as "secret," as they reflect well-known traditional spiritual and energetic (martial arts) practices.

Usui incorporated aspects of his Buddhist training into his Reiki teaching, including meditation, self-cleansing and a simple method of spiritual empowerment called Reiju, as well as some Shinto and Ki-kou energy practices. Although they are based on Buddhist and Shinto teachings, no specific religion is attached to them, so they are available to anyone, regardless of their religion or beliefs. (Buddhism is regarded as a way of life, rather than a religion.)

While originally Usui would simply sit in meditation with the students and transfer the Reiki energy connection across the room (in the way of a true spiritual master), he evidently found that a small ceremony was more useful for assisting the focus of some of his Shinpiden (level three) students, and also when there was a large group involved (empowerments are given on a one-to-one basis). This spiritual empowerment is what is now called Reiju, and although it may have been changed over time—and certainly the spiritual empowerments used in Western Reiki are more complex—it is used by the Gakkai in their training, and repeated each time a student attends a meeting.

It seems that Usui worked intuitively on people, placing his hands wherever he felt they were in need of healing. However, once he began to teach others to do Reiki he found that instructions were needed, and he wrote the *Usui Reiki Hikkei*, which was a two-part manual to be given to his students. This original Reiki manual has a section called Ryoho Shishon—"Guide to a Method of Healing." The purpose of the guide was to assist the Reiki practitioner who had not yet developed Byosen (the ability to feel where Reiki is required). The instructions include all the major body parts, as well as major illnesses that were common in Usui's time. Depending on the size of the treatment area, the practitioner could lay one or two hands on the area, or simply place their index and middle fingers on the area, because Reiki flows out of the fingertips as well as the palms of the hands.

USUI'S ORIGINAL HAND POSITIONS

It seems that Usui mainly concentrated on hand positions on the head, unless areas on the torso appeared to be out of balance energetically, apparently because the belief at that time was that most ailments arose in the brain. A number of different hand positions are in use today, although the 12 hand positions taught by Mrs. Takata do include four or five on the head, with seven or eight on the trunk of the body. These positions correspond to Eastern traditional teachings (such as Chinese Medicine) where the "body" is the head and torso, while the limbs are considered "external," and are therefore not normally treated. It is considered that applying healing energy to the head and thorax is sufficient to treat the whole body/mind.

The person receiving healing was usually seated, not lying down, and the healing began at the head. For a self-treatment there were five hand positions, all of which are illustrated in Chapter 10:

1. **Zento-bu** Top of the forehead, between the eyebrows and the line where the hair starts to grow.
2. **Koutou-bu** Back of the head, at the midpoint between the top of the head and the base of the skull.
3. **Enzui-bu** Base of the skull, where the brain and spine meet.
4. **Sokuto-bu** Both sides of the head, at the temples.
5. **Toucho-bu** Top of the head (the crown).

These positions are often combined into three hand positions when treating someone else, as shown below. The hand positions would be held for as long as necessary, but the total time would be about 30 minutes, after which other positions on the body would be treated— i.e., wherever an imbalance showed when the patient's energy field was scanned by the practitioner's hand(s).

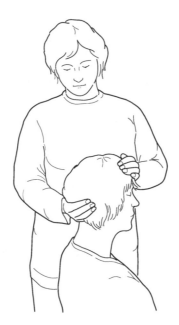

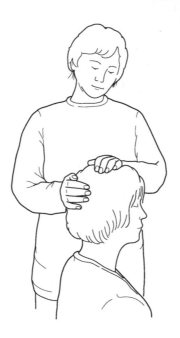

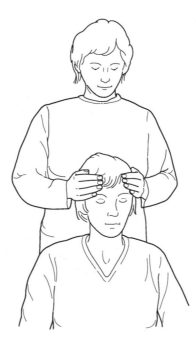

The first teachings (Shoden) are about "cleansing" (the use of hands-on healing, cleansing techniques, meditation and chanting of the Reiki principles) and "opening" (receiving of Reiju empowerment), for the healing of the Self.

The Inner (Okuden) and the Higher (Shinpiden) teachings take students further on their spiritual path, including—at a very much later stage—the learning of how to perform the Reiju empowerment ceremony. The importance of self-healing was imparted, as well as the benefits of living a "proper" life, using the Reiki principles as a foundation, which Usui is thought to have adopted from the Meiji emperor. Below is a version of these principles, which comes from an original document written by one of Usui's students (in Japanese kanji) with its translation into English. (Japanese text is read from right to left.)

招福の秘法
萬病の霊薬
今日丈けは 怒るな
心配すな 感謝して
業をはげめ 人に親切に
朝夕合掌して心に念じ
口に唱へよ
心身改善 臼井霊氣療法
肇祖
臼井甕男

The secret art of inviting happiness
The miraculous medicine of all diseases
Just for today, do not anger
Do not worry and be filled with gratitude
Devote yourself to your work and be kind to people
Every morning and evening join your hands in prayer,
Pray these words to your heart
And chant these words with your mouth
Usui Reiki treatment for the improvement of body and
   mind

The founder
Usui Mikao

In addition, Usui would advise his students to read 125 inspirational poems (Gyosei) from the Meiji emperor, in the Waka or Tanka style.

THE FOUNDING OF THE USUI REIKI RYOHO GAKKAI

Mikao Usui is also credited with founding the Usui Reiki Ryoho Gakkai (meaning the Usui Reiki Healing Method Learning Society), the organization dedicated to keeping the Reiki teachings alive, although it is probable that his followers started it after his death, naming Usui as the founder as a mark of respect. This society has continued to practice and teach Reiki in an unbroken line since 1926, the first few leaders being Shinpiden students taught by Usui, although they are not referred to as Grand Masters, but simply as Presidents of the Gakkai.

The Gakkai members follow Usui's teachings very closely,

and they hold regular meetings in Tokyo and elsewhere in Japan for their members, where the students read out Waka poetry, chant the Reiki principles, do Hatsurei-ho (a combined meditation and cleansing practice) and receive a Reiju empowerment from one of the Shinpiden members, for cleansing, purification and to strengthen their ability to access Reiki.

In 1999 a Japanese Reiki Master, Hiroshi Doi, visited Canada at the invitation of two of my Reiki Masters, Richard Rivard and Andy Bowling, and he taught a workshop on the Usui Reiki Ryoho, Usui's original system. He and some other Japanese Reiki Masters who are sympathetic toward sharing information with the West have helped us to understand much more about Usui's teachings.

SYNERGY

I hope you have found it useful and interesting to read about where Reiki came from, and how it has developed into the healing system we're familiar with today. Modern Reiki is in many ways still true to its Japanese spiritual traditions, although inevitably there have been some changes along the way. From Dr. Usui's experience of enlightenment, and his research into healing techniques from the Buddhist traditions, has come one of the world's most precious gifts—a holistic healing system that is easy to use and easy to learn. It connects us with a divinely guided energy to replenish our physical and energy bodies, and also helps us to develop personally and spiritually.

The original techniques that are still taught in Japan, and which are now beginning to be taught in the West, are a wonderful addition to everything we have learned through the Takata lineage, but of course we don't have to throw out the Western ideas. Much of what has been taught in the West for more than 50 years is still valid and useful, especially for people who are new to Reiki. Having a "formula" of 12 hand positions for Reiki treatments that is standard for every client (see Chapter 5) gives people something solid to work with, so that they can gradually develop their sensitivity. When they feel confident, they can use the more intuitive approach that is more common in Japan, and treat individuals according to their differing needs. Also, placing the hands in 12 positions evenly over the head and body allows the whole person to be treated. As well as creating balance, this also means that any areas that particularly need Reiki are treated automatically, whether the practitioner knows where the areas are or not, so it enables even the most inexperienced practitioner to produce consistent results.

In Part 2, I describe what it is like to receive a Reiki treatment, and what each hand position is treating, so that you have a better understanding of its benefits. I also explain the healing process, how Reiki works and how it contributes to the healing process, which I hope will intrigue and interest you enough to want to learn Reiki for yourself—and if so, that's what I deal with in Part 3.

part two

EXPERIENCING REIKI

chapter four

UNDERSTANDING THE HEALING PROCESS

In order to fully experience Reiki, you need to know about the healing process itself, what it is like to receive a treatment and what the effects and benefits are of doing so. Each of these aspects of Reiki is explained in the following three chapters.

In previous chapters I have described Reiki as a healing energy, and in the next few chapters I explain what it is like to receive a Reiki treatment, and say more about the effects receiving Reiki can have, and how it works. However, to begin with it is important to understand what healing is, and the ways in which energies impact on us.

AN INTRODUCTION TO ENERGY THEORY

To put it simply, everything in the universe is energy— this book, the chair I'm sitting on, the computer I'm using and my own physical body (and yours, of course!). Einstein and later quantum physicists have explained that at the quantum level—which is between 10,000 and

100,000 times smaller than an atom—everything that exists in the universe is energy, vibrating and oscillating at different rates. Recent studies of quantum physics have led to some fascinating discoveries, although scientists don't necessarily have any firm explanations, just theories. One theory is that all energy exists on a continuum from the most dense and least conscious, or what we call physical matter, to the least dense and most conscious, which we call spiritual.

Low Vibrations   **High Vibrations**
Dense Energy ←—————————→ **Spiritual Energy**
(Matter)   **(Consciousness)**

Science has finally caught up with thousands of years of spiritual teachings by proving that at the quantum level all energy—and therefore everything in the universe—is connected. Why is this of any interest to people learning Reiki? Because Reiki is a spiritual energy vibrating at a very high rate, and it works at an energetic level both with the physical matter of the body, and with the electromagnetic energy of the energy field that surrounds and interpenetrates the physical body. Understanding this will help you to understand why Reiki can help your healing on many different levels, from the physical to the mental, emotional and spiritual aspects of each individual.

HUMAN ENERGIES

The physical body is something we all know about—we can see it and feel it—yet every cell within it is actually energy or light, vibrating at a slow enough rate to make it into visible physical matter. The human body, and the energy field that surrounds and interpenetrates it, is made up of electromagnetic energy, and every person has a unique vibrational energy signature, or frequency, in the same way as we all have unique fingerprints, or DNA. We are familiar with the electromagnetic output of various parts of the body—the heart and brain, for example— being detected by scientific instruments, but the electromagnetic output of a person's whole body can also be measured using an electromyograph.

THE HUMAN ENERGY FIELD

The human energy field comprises both the physical body, which is energy or light vibrating at a slow enough rate to make it into visible physical matter, and an energy body that surrounds and interpenetrates it made up of much finer, lighter and higher vibrations which is more difficult to see. This energy body is made up of three parts:

1. **The aura** A field of electromagnetic energy with seven layers outside the physical body, of which our physical body is the innermost, densest layer.
2. **The chakras** A series of up to 20 active energy centers, the seven major chakras being located down the center of the physical body from the crown of the head to the perineum.
3. **The meridians** Lots of energy channels flowing throughout the body.

Perhaps the easiest way to understand this is to think of it in similar terms to parts of your physical body. The aura could be described as the energy equivalent of your whole physical body, the chakras could correspond to your brain, heart and other major organs, and the meridians are similar to your veins and arteries, but instead of blood, they carry energy—the life force we call Ki.

The energy that comprises the human energy field has various names, depending upon the culture or spiritual tradition—Ki (Japanese), Chi or Qi (Chinese), Prana (Indian), and Light or Holy Ghost (Christian), or it may simply be called life force. It flows within the physical body through the energy centers called chakras and energy pathways called meridians, as well as flowing around the body in the aura. When your Ki is high and flowing freely, you feel healthy, strong, confident, full of energy, and ready to enjoy life and take on its challenges, and you are much less likely to become ill. When your Ki is low, or there is a restriction or blockage in its flow, you feel weak, tired and lethargic, and are much more vulnerable to illness, or "dis-ease."

The Aura

The aura is a field of energy or light that completely surrounds the physical body above, below and on all sides. It is as much a part of you as your physical body, but the higher frequencies of the energies that make up the aura make it harder to see with the naked eye, although it can be detected by some scientific equipment, and a representation of the aura can be photographed using a special Kirlian camera. It is made up of seven layers, with the inner layers closest to the physical body comprising the

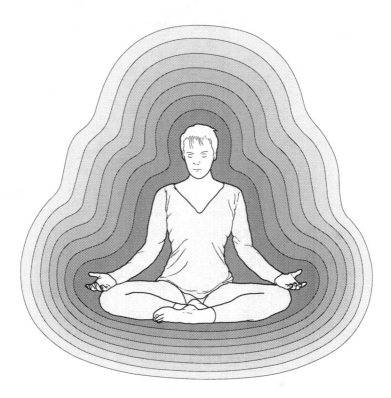

densest energy, and each succeeding layer being of finer and higher vibrations. Most people have an oval (elliptical) aura, which is slightly larger at the back than at the front, and fairly narrow at the sides, and it also stretches above the head and below the feet.

People's auras vary in size, but the outer edge of the aura can be anywhere between 1–2 meters (3–6 feet) from the physical body, to 20 meters (66 feet) or more in front of and behind the body. However, your aura doesn't stay the same size all the time, as it can expand or contract depending upon a variety of factors, such as how healthy you are, how you are feeling emotionally or psychologically at any given moment, or how comfortable you feel with the people in your immediate surroundings. This aura is spiritual energy, or Ki, which is present around each of us from birth (and before birth, as the fetus develops) until around the time of our death. Usually, just before death only a narrow band of spiritual energy remains, down what is referred to as the hara line, linking all the chakras in the center of the body, and shortly after physical death, no aura can be detected, because the Ki has returned to the Source (see page 92). However, in a living person the outer edges and the individual layers of the aura can be detected using dowsing rods or a pendulum, and they can also be sensed with the hands. With a little practice the densest layers, nearest to the body, can also be seen by most people with the naked eye, and some very psychic people can see the whole energy body quite clearly.

Although we may not be consciously aware of the fact, we all use our auras as valuable sensing devices—what you might call the "eyes in the back of your head." Have you ever experienced that strange "prickle" at the back of your neck when someone has been looking at you from behind? Or sensed an atmosphere even before you've entered a room? That's because your own aura extends 5 to 10 meters (15 to 30 feet) ahead of you, and behind you, so it is able to pick up the vibrations of other people's auras all around you.

ACTIVITY—SEEING YOUR AURA

◆ To see your own aura it is easiest to look at either (or both) of your hands. Hold your hand out at arm's length away from you, with the fingers spread wide apart, preferably with a plain background behind. Some people find it easiest with a light background, while others prefer something dark, so just experiment. What you are looking for is a faint misty outline close to and surrounding the fingers, which usually appears lighter than your finger color, although sometimes it is more like a slightly darker smudgy line.

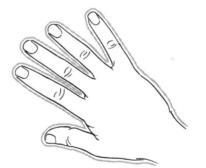

◆ It's important to be relaxed about this—a soft gaze is more likely to achieve results than a fiercely concentrated stare. If at first you don't succeed, try a different kind of background or better lighting—daylight is better than artificial light, and fluorescent lighting can make it particularly difficult. Also, don't expect to see masses of colored light: the auric field is usually softly colored, but it is very subtle, and is often "sensed" rather than seen.

♦ When you've successfully seen the aura around your own fingers, you might like to look for other people's auric fields. It is unusual to see auras all the time—most people "switch on" this ability by actively looking, so you're unlikely to notice them while wheeling your shopping cart around the supermarket! It is simplest when a person is involved in something important to them, such as giving an impassioned speech, because the aura seems to intensify at such times. It can be seen as a soft white or golden glow surrounding their head and shoulders, which grows larger as they become more involved in their subject. Again, it is probably best if they have a plain background behind them, but the more practice you have, the easier it gets, and eventually you will probably begin to see (or sense) shades of other colors, too. If you are interested in learning more about auras and what can be detected in them, see page 287 for recommended books.

Some people develop a particular skill in "reading" auras, and they are sometimes called "medical intuitives," because they can detect illnesses and imbalances within the aura, often before they have actually manifested in the physical body. The most famous medical intuitive is Caroline Myss, and I can highly recommend her book *Anatomy of the Spirit* on this subject.

The Chakras

Chakra is a Sanskrit word meaning "wheel," "disk" or "vortex," and very intuitive people describe the chakras as funnel-shaped energy, similar to a tornado or whirlpool, with the narrowest point near the body, and the widest point 30–60 centimeters (1–2 feet) away from the body. The chakras are energy centers at various points around the energy body where the spiritual energy of your aura, the Ki, or life force, circulates actively. There are seven major chakras in the human body, located on an energetic line running down the center of the body, called the hara line. They are at: 1) the perineum, near the base of the

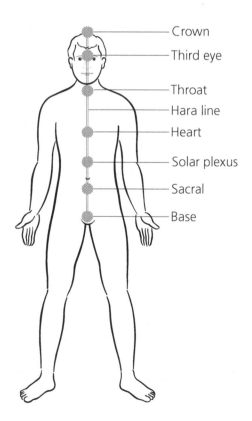

Crown

Third eye

Throat

Hara line

Heart

Solar plexus

Sacral

Base

The Seven Major Chakras

Chakra	Location	Color	Body parts/systems
7 Crown	Top of Head	Purple or Violet or White	Pineal/Pituitary, Nervous System, Brain, and Whole Body
6 Brow (Third Eye)	Center of Forehead	Indigo	Pituitary/Pineal, Hypothalamus, Endocrine System, Head, Eyes, Face
5 Throat	Throat	Blue	Thyroid, Parathyroid, Growth, Metabolism, Ears, Nose, Mouth, Teeth, Neck, Throat
4 Heart	Center of Chest (Sternum)	Green (sometimes pink)	Thymus, Respiration, Circulation, Immune System, Heart, Lungs, Upper Back, Arms, Hands
3 Solar Plexus	Solar Plexus	Yellow	Pancreas, Muscles, Digestive System, Liver, Gall Bladder, Middle Back
2 Sacral	Abdomen (Navel)	Orange	Testes/Ovaries, Reproduction System, Kidneys, Uterus, Lower Digestive Organs, Lower Back
1 Root or Base	Base of Spine	Red	Adrenals, Skeleton, Skin, Elimination System, Senses, Pelvis, Hips, Legs, Feet

Associated life aspects	Chant/note
Knowledge, Spirituality, Understanding, Unity, Connection, Universal Consciousness **I Know**	EE Top "C"
Clairvoyance, Intuition, Imagination, Spiritual Awareness, Individual Consciousness **I See**	AY "B"
Communication, Expression, Creativity, Abundance, Receiving **I Speak**	I (EYE) "A"
Unconditional Love, Balance, Unity, Relationships, Affinity, Giving, Acceptance **I Love**	AH "G"
Personal Power, Will, Control, Self-Definition, Energy, Intellect **I Can**	OH "F"
Emotions, Sensations, Sexuality, Food, Appetite, Movement, Pleasure **I Feel**	OOH "E"
Survival, Security, Trust, Grounding, Physical Body, Money, Home, Job **I Have**	URGH "D"

spine, 2) near the navel, 3) at the solar plexus, 4) in the middle of the chest, 5) in the throat, 6) at the center of the brow, and 7) on the crown of the head. In addition there are a number of minor chakras, for instance in the palms of the hands, on the knees and on the soles of the feet.

Each chakra is linked to one layer of the aura. The base chakra is linked to the auric layer closest to the body, the sacral chakra to the second layer, the solar plexus to the third layer, and so on. A healthy chakra vibrates evenly in a circular motion, either clockwise or counterclockwise, and this can be detected by using a pendulum held over the chakra point (or sometimes people can actually feel the energy moving with their hands), and the outer edge can be only a few inches from the body or several feet away, depending upon the person's physical, mental and emotional state. Chakras are intimately connected to our physical health, as each is linked with specific parts of the body, and to systems within the body. When a particular chakra is healthy, balanced and open, so are its connected body parts, but when a chakra is blocked, damaged or too closed, the health of the connected body parts and systems will begin to reflect this. Our chakras are affected by everything that happens to us— good things as well as bad. For example, falling in love has an amazingly beneficial effect on our whole energy body, whereas emotional or mental traumas, and even negative words, can have detrimental effects on the energy levels.

A chakra can be described as open, closed, or at any of the various stages in between, basically reflecting a person's personality or a reaction to a particular situation.

For example, a chakra may be fully open when someone is feeling very happy or safe, or closed when they are feeling ill or threatened, but a blocked chakra may be unable to change its state easily, being "stuck" in either an open or closed state, which will affect the general flow of Ki around the physical and energy bodies, and thereby the general state of health of the person. The chakra then needs healing, to uncover and remove whatever is blocking it. If you are attuned to Reiki you can use it to clear blockages in that area, and it is also important to take steps to change the patterns of behavior responsible for the block. However, a blockage in one chakra can influence the activity of the ones above and below it—so, for example, you may have problems with self-esteem and personal power (third chakra), but this could be influenced by your feelings about sex (second chakra), whereas the real problem may be that you find it difficult to love yourself unconditionally (fourth chakra).

The Meridians

These are the tiny energy lines which carry life-force energy around the whole physical body, connecting all parts of the body to the chakra system. For example, during an acupuncture treatment the meridian points (where the meridians touch the skin) are stimulated by needles to help to clear blockages. However, during a Reiki treatment the meridians carry the Reiki energy around the whole human energy system (and be reassured, no needles are used!).

Perhaps you can now see that there is a connection between energy and healing, especially where Reiki is concerned.

Your aura and chakras have been regulating themselves quite naturally all your life, but now that you are aware of them you can help yourself by carrying out the visualization at the end of this chapter. It will help to cleanse your aura, and balance, clear and harmonize your chakras, leaving you relaxed yet alert and ready to face the day.

YOUR LIFE-FORCE ENERGY—KI

Your aura and the rest of your energy body constitute your life-force energy, or Ki, and the idea that this energy exists has been part of the wisdom of most cultures around the world for thousands of years.

However, the amount of Ki within us varies from day to day—there is a natural rhythmic ebb and flow in the energies within our bodies—but we absorb Ki in a variety of ways in order to "top off" our supply, because clearly we use some of it every day. The most obvious form in which we take in Ki is through food and drink, because all animal and plant life, and even water, is filled with this Ki, too.

As well as taking in Ki from the food we eat, we also breathe it in, and absorb it through our aura, as Ki energy is everywhere—it is the connective force of the universe— so there is a limitless supply. However, the amount of Ki we absorb is not constant, and can depend on many factors, so we don't always sufficiently replenish our supply. If this happens over a long period of time our energy body can become too depleted, so we become weaker and more susceptible to illness and the aging process, and even physical death—because your Ki is what defines you as a living being; without it you would not be alive.

The levels of Ki in our bodies have an impact on our inherent healing ability, as Ki helps to nourish the structure, organs and systems of the body, supporting them in their vital functions and contributing to the healthy growth and renewal of cells.

Healthy young children usually take in as much Ki as they need in this natural way—you only have to watch them running about to see that their energy levels are high. People who study ancient spiritual practices, special breathing techniques or martial arts are also often able to focus additional energy and draw it into their bodies. However, the rest of us, particularly as we get older, may not draw in as much Ki as we need, and therefore our reserves become depleted. You may have experienced this yourself occasionally, for instance when you have spent time with a friend who is going through some emotionally traumatic event. Usually after a few hours of talking supportively to them you begin to feel drained and tired, and this is because you have "donated" your Ki, or have allowed it to be drawn off into your friend's energy field, because you have acknowledged on a subconscious level their greater need.

This is one way in which we are all able to "heal," by using our own Ki for the benefit of others. Other examples are when we cuddle a child to stop it from crying, or place a hand on a cut or painful part of the body. At this level, we may not think of ourselves as "healers," but we are helping our own or another person's healing process by using our personal supply of Ki energy.

WHAT IS HEALING?

The dictionary definition of the word "healing" is "to restore or be restored to health." Most people seem to think of healing as something that happens "out there"—that some-one else "heals" them, whether that other person is a doc-tor, a therapist or a practitioner of a complementary therapy. But there is only one "healer" in your life, and that is *you*.

Consider for a moment what happens when you cut yourself—I mean after you've said "Ouch!" washed the cut and put a Band-Aid on it! The cut doesn't continue to bleed, or remain open for the rest of your life—it heals up, doesn't it? So who heals it? You do. Your body has all the healing power it needs, and that healing is activated when something goes wrong. Think of every time you've had the "common cold." No matter what medications you choose to take for it, from a simple aspirin to one of the more complex preparations that seek to reduce your symptoms for at least 12 hours, there is no known "cure" for a cold. It is a virus that has beaten scientists for many years. But your body gets rid of it. Your immune system is mobilized, and usually within a few days you are feeling healthy again—and indeed, it is your body's reaction to the virus that gives you all of those nasty symptoms, such as a runny nose and a tickly cough.

Of course you may question this assumption of being able to heal yourself when you think of serious illnesses such as cancer, but there are many reported cases of people who have healed themselves of life-threatening diseases, sometimes with astonishing speed. However, they have usually used something to help them to acti-vate their own healing ability—it might have been positive thinking, visualizations, meditation, Reiki or one of any number of complementary therapies—and to help to mobilize their body's defenses. Even with the intervention of surgery or medication it is still the physical body that heals itself, as it knits together cut flesh or utilizes the chemicals to reduce symptoms, or produce different effects (although all drugs have side effects, and most simply suppress or change the body's chemical balance, rather than actually curing the problem).

So healing is a very personal thing, but universally people still think of it as being healing at a physical level, whereas the reality is much wider, encompassing mind, emotions and spirit, as well as the physical body.

Expanding the Definition

An increasing number of people involved in health care now believe that treating the physical body without healing the other aspects of the self (the mental, emotional and spiritual) is like putting a patch on a burst tire. It may help for a while, but it should be viewed as a temporary solution while you look for the cause. Otherwise the problem will simply occur again, either in the same form or as some new disease, until the message that the body is trying to bring to you is heeded and there is a change in consciousness—in the way you think and behave. "Healing" in this expanded sense is the realization that you have a direct and important role to play in activating your own vibrant health; that you have some choice in the matter. You can choose to help yourself, whether by adopting a healthier lifestyle or by deciding what healing needs to take place and seeking ways to bring this about.

Of course, many things can impact your body's natural healing ability:

- ◆ Whether you eat a healthy balanced diet.
- ◆ Whether you drink plenty of water.
- ◆ Whether you get sufficient sleep.
- ◆ Whether you are too tired or under a great deal of stress.
- ◆ Your age and general state of health, and so on.

For example, poor nutrition reduces healing rates and increases susceptibility to infection, which further delays healing, and studies have also proved that psychological stress has a similar delaying effect on the body's healing processes.

All Healing is Self-healing

So good health isn't just something that occurs automatically, regardless of what you do, and healing isn't something that happens "out there," something that someone else "does" to you. No matter from whom you seek help for your healing, whether it is a doctor, nurse or complementary therapist, and no matter what interventions they might suggest, from medicines to herbal remedies, surgery to massage, there is really only one "healer" of your body, and that is *you*. Your body possesses the mechanisms to heal itself, so all anyone else can do is to help that natural process in some way.

The Difference between Healing and Curing

That brings us to another topic—the relationship between healing and curing. Many people use the words "healing" and "curing" interchangeably, yet they don't necessarily mean the same thing. *Curing* means completely eradicating an illness or disease, whereas *healing* can occur on many different levels, and doesn't have to be linked with a physical illness at all.

1. Healing on the **physical** level. This might mean eradicating an illness completely, or it could simply mean limiting or alleviating the symptoms for a time while you learn about and tackle any causative issues on the emotional, mental or spiritual levels.
2. Healing on the **emotional** level. This could allow you to calm any fears and to reach an acceptance of the effects of the illness, or help you to come to terms with loss or bereavement, or allow you to let go of destructive emotions such as anger, jealousy and resentment.
3. Healing on the **mental** (psychological) level. This could enable you to think differently about your illness, perhaps bringing to your attention the lessons your illness is trying to teach, and promoting understanding of the causative issues; or it could help you to let go of destructive, negative thought patterns, attitudes or prejudices that are holding you back.
4. Healing on the **spiritual** level. This could enable you to develop a more loving and forgiving relationship with yourself, helping you to achieve greater self-esteem; or it could help you to let go of belief systems that are restricting you, allowing you greater self-expression and creativity; or perhaps even help you at the end of your life to make a peaceful transition into death.

On a physical level, however, let me give you one graphic example to demonstrate the difference there can be between healing and curing. In the case of someone who is unfortunate enough to develop gangrene in their foot or lower leg, it may be necessary to amputate the leg below the knee in order to *cure* the illness—and hopefully, if the disease has been caught in time, the gangrene will indeed be eradicated, and in practical terms the body's natural processes will then be activated to heal the wound caused by the operation.

However, an amputation certainly does not *heal* the person, because such an operation will have an enormous psychological, emotional and even spiritual impact upon that person, from the way they view themselves and come to terms with their new body image, to their relationships with other people. Will they still feel loved and attractive, or will they expect or receive rejection from others? What will be the impact on their everyday lives? Can they cope with the challenges to mobility or dexterity that the loss of a limb can cause? What about their future aims, ambitions and potential? Will they learn to live with any restriction and find new outlets for their talents, or will they believe life is simply not worth living anymore?

THE BODY/MIND CONNECTION

If you go to the doctor complaining about an upset stomach or painful joints, the doctor's trained response is to give you something to deal with the symptom, but little or no attention is usually paid to the cause. The cause may be something purely physical—you may have eaten something that has disagreed with you, or strained a joint through some physical activity—but although those are fairly uncomplicated examples, there may be something other than purely physical reasons going on.

The discovery that the mind can affect the body is seen as something relatively recent, but actually most ancient forms of treatment, such as Ayurvedic or Chinese medicine, are based on the mind/body connection. Scientists can now explain the connection in a simple way— wherever thought or emotion goes, a chemical goes with it. For example, fear triggers the "fight or flight" response and releases the hormone adrenaline; happiness floods the system with endorphins, which make us feel good, and also produce the benefit of fitting into the body's pain receptors and therefore blocking the pain signals to the brain so we don't feel it so much.

BODY WISDOM

There are many people (and I'm one of them) who believe that your body has its own form of consciousness, and that at all times, under all circumstances, your body is trying to be your loving and helpful friend. Every ache or pain, discomfort or disease, illness or imbalance is your body's way of conversing with you. It is always in direct contact with your Higher Self (your Soul or Spirit), in ways in which your conscious mind is not, and your Higher Self, through the medium of your body, uses the solid, physical aspects of yourself to give you messages. Your Higher Self has total, unconditional love for your Whole Self and for your

Physical Self, and always wants what is best for you, and if you are in some way "off track," or doing things (or even thinking or saying things) that are harmful to you in some way, it uses your body to try to get a message to you, to bring something to your attention. The more "in tune" with your body wisdom you become, the faster (and simpler) the messages become.

I do try to "tune in" to my body, and to understand what is going on, so I often get quick, easy messages. The most common are reactions to negative thoughts or an inability to make a decision, "worrying" the decision over in my mind. In these cases I tend to get sudden pains in my knee, ankle or foot—all dealing with "where I am going." These are almost always on the left side of my body, which is more directly concerned with my spiritual journey through life, although if I am thinking negatively about money, or other issues of physical security, then it will be my right leg that reacts, or I might get an ache in my lower back. After my initial reaction of "Ouch!" the stab of pain is enough to make me stop and pay proper attention to whatever I have been thinking about, rather than just letting thoughts idly float around my mind. It directs me to "mindfulness," creating awareness of the present moment, making me pause and just "be" for a while, to let my thought processes slow down so that I can eliminate the negativity or indecision.

REACTING TO THE MESSAGES

Most people react to illness or disease by trying to get rid of the symptoms as quickly as possible, usually by seeking medical advice or intervention, and that's a natural enough reaction. No one wants to feel ill. However, a recent advertisement on television caught my attention, because it was extolling the virtues of a popular analgesic as something "for people who don't have time to have headaches." From my perspective this attitude is quite alarming, because while there is nothing wrong in seeking relief for symptoms, if you really want your body to be healed, you also need to understand the illness at the causative level, and if you have constant headaches, "masking" them with medication and carrying on as if nothing was wrong isn't a long-term solution. You're not listening to what your body is trying to tell you, so although the symptoms might abate briefly they will return because you are not taking your body's advice and acting upon it.

Your first priority is therefore to ask yourself "*Why* am I ill?" From this metaphysical perspective, illness or disease is created by the body—or the body/mind connection— as a helpful message, an indication that there is an imbalance somewhere. As the body is simply a part of our consciousness this means that we actually create our own ill health. There have been many experiments that have shown that the mind can create symptoms, such as a study carried out on a group of children who all knew they were allergic to poison ivy. While blindfolded, the children were told that poison ivy was being brushed against their skin—although in fact a totally innocuous plant was being used—and each one almost immediately produced red and blistered skin where the plant had touched them. Their *belief* that the plant would produce a reaction actually caused their body to react as if it was real. So the idea that your mind works with your body to produce illness and disease may be a very challenging concept, but really it is very empowering, because if between them your mind and body have the power to create ill health, then they also have the power to create good health.

TAKING RESPONSIBILITY FOR YOUR OWN WELL-BEING

It is important not to take the above on board as some kind of "blame theory." Although from this perspective you may be responsible at a deep and unconscious mind/body connection level for having created an illness, this isn't being done at a conscious level, so there is no blame attached, and you therefore should not judge yourself—or anyone else—harshly for being ill. You don't suddenly wake up one morning and say, "Oh, I think I'll break my leg today—that'll stop me rushing around doing too much and I can have a good rest and some time to think about my direction in life!" or, "Hmm, I've got a lot of suppressed emotion and anger and resentment inside me, so I think I'll let my body develop cancer or heart disease to give me a message I can't ignore." Of course not! From a human perspective that would be utter madness. But from a Soul/Higher Self level the destructive ability of the cancer or the pain of the broken leg are simply experiences on your journey through this physical life. If you heed the messages, all well and good, and you can heal and move on; if you don't they will lead to different life experiences, so again from the Soul perspective that is still okay. *You are a spiritual being having a physical experience, not a physical being having a spiritual experience!*

These theories may be pretty difficult to come to terms with if you haven't heard them before, and they may well challenge your belief system or your concept of how the world works. Of course, you are free to take them on board or ignore them—the choice is yours. But if reading about them has sparked at least an interest in finding out more then there are some recommended books in Further Reading (see page 287) that you might find useful. Having challenged you somewhat, let me introduce a calming, relaxing inner journey that I hope you will find enjoyable. It takes you through a visualization of the seven major chakras, and bathes them in beautiful, soothing color.

ACTIVITY—VISUALIZATION

Preparing for the Visualization

You will find it easiest to meditate or visualize if you are in a safe, quiet, softly lit environment where disturbances will be as few as possible. You may like to create a special place in your home where you can sit or lie down in comfort, and the experience may be enhanced if you are able to burn some favorite essential oils or incense sticks, and perhaps have some gentle music playing softly in the background.

◆ Two great tools to aid meditation are relaxation and breathing control, and as part of the process of meditation you might like to develop the habit of relaxing your body by visualizing and feeling it relax.

◆ First, feel your feet on the floor, then tense the muscles of your toes, feet and heels and relax them completely. Next, tense the muscles of your calves, knees and thighs, and then let them relax. Then tense the muscles of your hips, abdomen and chest, and let them relax, and slow your breathing to an even rate. Finally, tense and then relax the muscles of your shoulders, arms, hands and fingers, and your neck, jaw, face and scalp.

◆ This method is good because most of us tend to store a lot of tension, particularly in our shoulders and legs, so you might like to tense and relax those areas three or four times. When you're feeling relaxed—and with practice this will take only two or three minutes—become aware of your breathing. Perhaps count the breaths and allow yourself to fall into a slow, regular pattern of breathing, and then you can begin the visualization.

◆ If you haven't tried visualizations before, don't worry about the process. We are all used to imagining things, or daydreaming, or remembering things, and that's all that visualizing is, on a practical level. It is using your imagination to take you on a journey in your mind, and if you are not a particularly visual person then you may just sense what is happening—and that is fine. However, try to remember, with your eyes closed, what your bedroom looks like. Can you "see" it? Well, that's visualizing! If you see a few dissociated images, or you complete only part of the visualization, or get some of the sights, sounds or smells, or an outline without any detail, then just take whatever comes. You can always return to the visualization at another time, and indeed you can repeat it again and again if you want to, and gradually the fuller picture will develop.

◆ Each of the main chakras "vibrates" to a particular color, as given below, and part of this visualization takes you through a rainbow of light, which helps to open, clear and balance each chakra, enabling Ki to flow more effectively through you. If you think visualizing a color might be a challenge, then try "seeing" a red rose, or an orange, a lemon, some green grass, a summery blue sky, a pair of dark denim jeans and some sumptuous purple velvet. That can make it much easier.

Chakra Colors—Bringing In the Light

◆ Sit in a comfortable position and allow your body to relax. Begin to be aware of your breathing, and follow your breath in and out, in and out; with each breath you are becoming more and more relaxed. Now imagine that you are breathing in beautiful bright white light, and see or feel this brilliant light swirling around, filling your head, and with every inward breath the light flows into more of your body. It flows down into your neck, shoulders and arms, moving right down into your hands to the very tips of your fingers. Then you see or sense it flowing through your back and chest, and down into your abdomen, and then into your thighs, knees and down into your calves, ankles and feet, right to the tips of your toes. You feel your feet becoming heavier and more solid, and you can feel the connection with the floor beneath you, and then allow the white light to flow out of your feet into the earth. Imagine the white light forming roots growing from your feet down into the earth, anchoring you and making you feel very secure.

◆ Now the whole of your body is flooded with white light, you can use this light to form a protective barrier around you. Imagine that the light is coming out of your hands and visualize yourself moving your hands over all of your body so that a cloak of white light surrounds you until the whole of your aura is filled with white light. Now allow that light to spread out even further, filling the room, and watch the light swirl into all the corners, from floor to ceiling, from wall to wall, from door to window, until the whole room is bathed in protective white light.

◆ Then take your attention back to your body, and allow the white light to slowly change color until you are breathing in warm red light. Allow this red light to flow down and down your body until it reaches your root chakra at the base of your spine. Feel the red light clearing and balancing your root chakra, then sense it spreading out to fill the lower part of your body, and see it flowing down your legs and into your feet. You can even see it flowing down into the roots of light you have created into the earth.

◆ With your next breath you see the light changing to vibrant orange, and you allow this light to flow down your body until it reaches your sacral chakra, near your navel, and you feel the orange light clearing and balancing your sacral chakra, and then spreading out to fill all of that part of your body.

◆ Now allow yourself to breathe in golden yellow light, and see this yellow light flow down your body until it reaches your solar plexus, spreading out to clear and balance your solar plexus chakra.

◆ Next the light changes to a lovely soft green, and this green light flows down into your chest, where it clears, balances and harmonizes your heart chakra, and as it does so it spreads out to fill the whole of your chest, flowing also down your arms and into your hands, until even your fingers are filled with this lovely green light.

◆ The light now changes to a beautiful bright blue, and this blue light fills your throat and neck, and you see it swirling around, clearing and balancing your throat chakra.

◆ Your next breath brings in a deeper, indigo blue light, and this light flows up into your head, swirling around your brow chakra, and you sense it clearing and balancing your third eye.

◆ Finally you see the light you are breathing in change to a beautiful violet or purple, and this light flows up to the top of your head, where it clears and balances your crown chakra, and you sense that chakra opening like the petals of a flower, allowing the violet light to stream out, tinting your aura with its delicate rays.

◆ Then just enjoy the peace and tranquility of your protected space, and allow any stray thoughts that come into your mind to simply drift across, and remain in a relaxed, meditative state for five or ten minutes, or as long as you feel is comfortable. Whenever you are ready, gently become aware again of your surroundings, stretch your fingers and toes, allow your eyes to open, and feel refreshed and alert.

chapter five

RECEIVING A REIKI TREATMENT

Most people's first contact with Reiki is through receiving a Reiki treatment. This may be from a friend or relative who has just been on a Reiki course and wants someone to practice on, or it might be from a professional Reiki practitioner working in their own home or in a holistic therapy center or beauty salon. In either case, it will be from someone who has received the ability to channel the Reiki through their hands, and who has learned the specific hand positions to enable the Reiki to flow most easily throughout the body.

Reiki is a beautifully simple technique that requires no special medicines or equipment, and a Reiki treatment is a very relaxing experience for most people. Taking about an hour, treatments are generally carried out with your remaining fully clothed (except for shoes) and tucked up comfortably with a blanket and pillows, usually on a massage table. The practitioner's hands are placed and held still for a few minutes—there is no pressure, manipulation or massage—in specific positions over your head and body, working over the chakras (see Chapter 4) or areas of specific pain. As the energy flows through, you are able to achieve a very deep state of relaxation (many people fall asleep during the treatment), which allows physical, mental or emotional stress to leave the body, and the Reiki usually alleviates physical pain or discomfort and promotes a general feeling of well-being.

The Reiki energy makes its own way to the areas of the person's body, mind and spirit most in need of treatment. Sometimes people report beautiful dreams or visions, memories or colors arising during a treatment, and most experience a wonderful, glowing radiance afterward. At times there may be an emotional release— an urge to laugh or cry—or you may find that your limbs suddenly jerk even while you are asleep, but this is perfectly normal: it is just energy releasing in different ways from the body. Occasionally there will be temporary physical symptoms such as a sudden cold in the days immediately following a treatment, as the energy works through the blockages, releasing the physical, mental or emotional toxins, and the body does its best to get rid of them in the most efficient way. It is also possible that after a treatment you may experience a shift in consciousness, a realization of the causes of the problems—this is an important part of healing, and if you feel you would like to discuss this with your practitioner, they will respect your need for confidentiality.

Most people who go for a Reiki treatment want help with a specific physical problem, from frequent headaches or a frozen shoulder, to more long-term complaints such as chronic back pain or immune-system disorders, although some simply want to be able to relax and cope better with the stresses of modern life. Many physical symptoms are eased very quickly, while others, especially chronic conditions, may need a lot of Reiki before starting to respond—but as I explained in Chapter 4, it is your own body that has to do the healing, and while some people report amazing, even miraculous, effects, these cannot be guaranteed. Indeed, if there were ten people with identical physical symptoms having an identical number of Reiki treatments from the same practitioner, there would be ten different results, because each person is unique, and their physical, emotional, psychological and spiritual needs would not be the same.

While the potential with Reiki is unlimited, we often place limits on our own healing by what we believe is or is not possible. However, it is important to understand that whatever your expectations are of the outcome of a Reiki treatment, the Reiki will flow through you to unblock the causative level of disease (i.e., a lack of balance or harmony). While your conscious mind might think help with a physical symptom is the priority, it is your Higher Self which draws the Reiki into you, that part of you which knows what the underlying metaphysical causes are, whether emotional, mental or spiritual, so healing may need to take place on that level first. If, therefore, you've got a painful, stiff knee, you may get some relief for the knee, but the underlying metaphysical cause might have something to do with decisions you are finding difficult to make about your progress through life. So if you are willing to receive the Reiki, healing will take place, although it might not be quite what you expect. (Belief in Reiki is not a prerequisite—it also works well on animals, and of course they don't know what it is.)

WHO CAN BE TREATED?

The short answer is anyone, whatever their age, gender, ethnic group, religion or any other demographic classification to which they might belong. Babies and small children usually love to receive Reiki, although they don't often want to stay still long enough for a full treatment, and since they are so much smaller than adults they don't need as much anyway—it is far easier for them to be treated casually by allowing Reiki to flow while the practitioner holds them or when they sit on the therapist's knee. Older children and teenagers either seem to be wildly enthusiastic about Reiki, or rather suspicious, but once they have the opportunity to receive some, they usually like it. Pregnant women normally find Reiki to be very soothing for themselves and their unborn child, and it can be really beneficial to both mother and baby to receive Reiki during the birth process, if they are fortunate enough to have a family member or close friend who practices Reiki. Elderly people also find it very helpful with all the aches and pains that old age seems to bring—my mother took a Reiki course at the age of 80 so that she could treat herself and the other residents in the sheltered housing where she lived.

HOW MANY TREATMENTS?

This is rather like asking, "How long is a piece of string?" and it clearly depends upon what is being treated. For minor health problems or to alleviate stress and encourage relaxation, one or two treatments may be enough, while major illnesses are likely to require many treatments. For very serious or chronic conditions it is generally accepted that receiving four treatments, preferably on consecutive days, is an extremely effective way to start any treatment program, as it allows the Reiki to flow especially well through each of the four energy bodies—physical, emotional, mental and spiritual. If it isn't possible to attend treatments on four consecutive days, then at least two sessions per week for two weeks would be ideal, after which one a week would probably suffice until the problem is alleviated. One treatment each month is a good way to continue the healing as part of a maintenance program.

Another recommendation for dealing with serious illness is for the affected person to receive a full treatment every day for at least 21 days. This is obviously easier to achieve if a member of your own family or a friend who lives locally practices Reiki, but in other cases a combination of "hands-on" and distant treatments from a practitioner can be given, if the practitioner has acquired the skills taught at the second level of training (see Chapter 7).

WHAT TO EXPECT BEFORE THE TREATMENT

Reiki can be used without any equipment at all, because all the practitioner really needs is a pair of hands. However, most practitioners will carry out their Reiki treatments on a massage table, usually covered by a fitted sheet, and pillows and a soft blanket will also be offered.

Some practitioners work in holistic therapy centers or beauty salons, others have a room set aside in their home, while some offer a mobile service, taking a portable massage table to a client's home. If you find it difficult to lie flat for any reason, either on your back or on your front, it is quite possible to receive a treatment while lying on your side or sitting in a chair—do feel free to discuss this with your practitioner; don't just put up with being uncomfortable.

Before the treatment starts, you should have the opportunity to talk to the practitioner about your reasons for wanting it. If it is your first treatment, some basic medical details will also be taken, such as present or previous medical conditions, and any medication you are currently taking, as well as your name, date of birth, address, telephone number, and so on, and you should be reassured that this information will be kept confidential. The practitioner should also explain to you what they will be doing during the treatment, for instance where on your body their hands will be placed, so that this doesn't come as a surprise, and you have the chance to object if need be. However, as you can see from the diagrams later in this chapter, there is *never* any need for the therapist's hands to be placed on any intimate areas of the body— the breasts or genitals, for example—even if you have a condition that needs to be treated in those areas. Reiki will flow into those areas from nearby (above or below the breasts, or on the hip bones, for example), or the practitioner can hold their hands several inches above any areas you would not wish to be touched. This is also the case if you have any parts of your body that are too sore to be touched—with burns or bad cuts, for example. You remain fully clothed during a Reiki treatment (although coats and shoes should be removed), and this usually helps people to feel more confident and secure.

The practitioner will almost certainly do their best to make you feel comfortable, safe and supported before, during and after your treatment, and if you are attending their premises you should find them clean and welcoming. You may be asked to take off your watch and any metal jewelry (except for wedding rings), as there is a slight possibility that these could interfere with the flow of Reiki, or get caught by the practitioner's hands during the treatment.

Many therapists like to play gentle music in the background, usually classical or "new age" music, but you should be asked first if this is acceptable to you. Similarly, some practitioners like to burn an incense stick, or perhaps some lavender oil in a burner, but your permission to do this should be sought first, and if you have any difficulties with breathing, such as asthma, make them clear to the practitioner when you make your appointment so that oils or incense are not used immediately before your arrival, as these conditions can be aggravated by smoke or scents. Most practitioners are aware that they shouldn't wear perfume when treating clients, for the same reason, but if any particular perfumes irritate you, make this known to them as well. Talking or asking questions during the treatment is an individual matter, but being quiet allows you to relax more thoroughly, although of course if you are uncomfortable at any stage during the treatment, do speak out.

Before the actual treatment starts, the practitioner may carry out some personal preparation, such as meditating for a few minutes, and may do some energy cleansing on themselves and on you, which is quite pleasant, and normally involves them drawing their hands in the air around your body, in front, behind and on either side, so this often takes place with you sitting on a chair, or standing (see illustration below). (For more information about energy cleansing, see Chapter 11.)

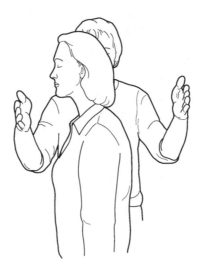

The practitioner may also "scan" in the air surrounding your body with one or both hands before the treatment begins, and after it has finished, which is a technique where they assess the energetic "feel" of your aura. This can help to identify areas that need more Reiki during the treatment, and whether those areas have cleared after the treatment. Again, this is often a pleasant activity, and usually takes place when you are lying on the massage table, although it, too, can be carried out with you sitting on a chair or standing.

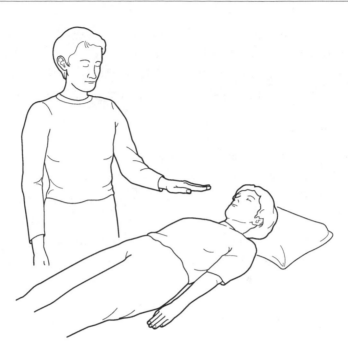

TREATMENT HAND POSITIONS

A full Reiki treatment usually comprises four or five hand positions on the head, four on the front of the body, and four on the back of the body, each traditionally held for about five minutes, although the timing of individual positions may vary. This is because the practitioner will be aware of the Reiki flowing through their hands, and will be able to assess whether or not the flow of Reiki has reduced earlier—say, after three minutes, indicating that it is time to move the hands to the next position. Alternatively, if the Reiki is still flowing strongly at the end of five minutes, they may decide to leave their hands longer on any position, as this often means that this particular area needs more attention.

There will also be some minor variations in the hand positions, depending obviously on how the practitioner was taught, and some practitioners also treat the legs and feet as well as the head and body, while others don't ask the client to turn over for the back positions, but treat the front of the body for longer. Whichever way the treatment is carried out, however, and regardless of how many hand positions are used, the Reiki will flow around the whole body, and so all areas will be treated at all levels—physically, emotionally, mentally and spiritually.

It is usual for the treatment to start with you lying on your back (unless you have discussed your needs with your practitioner and decided another position would be more comfortable for you) with one or more pillows under your head and also under your knees, and with the practitioner standing or sitting behind your head for the first few hand positions. Their hands will rest very gently on your fully clothed body, but if you ever feel the pressure is too much, please do say so. The practitioner will then move to the side of the table for the remaining hand positions, and you will often be gently encouraged to turn onto your tummy for the hand positions on your back; the position of the pillows will be changed to underneath your ankles, which helps to take the strain off your back. This part of the treatment can also be carried out with you lying on your side.

HAND POSITIONS FOR THE HEAD

There are a number of ways in which a practitioner may start the Reiki treatment, and each is equally valid—as I explain in later chapters, the way practitioners are trained does vary, and some develop their own style of treatment after some years of experience, so you don't need to worry if the descriptions of any of the hand placements differ from those you experience. Provided you are comfortable, that's fine, but if any hand position makes you feel nervous or uncomfortable (if the practitioner's hands are too close to your throat, for example) then ask them to move their hands until it feels acceptable for you. For each hand position I have given an explanation of what is potentially being treated at a physical level, because I will deal with other aspects in Chapter 6.

Three main hand positions can be used to begin treatment, and doing any of these in any order is quite satisfactory.

1. One hand underneath the client's head and the other hand resting on the crown of the client's head. This position is sometimes used to start a special type of treatment designed to work deeply on psychological or emotional issues.

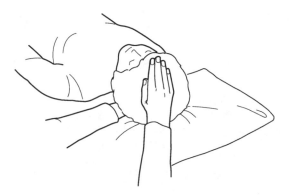

2. Both hands underneath the client's head.

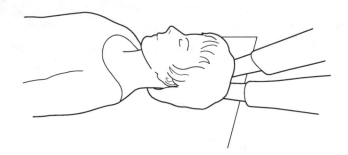

3. Both hands over the client's eyes.

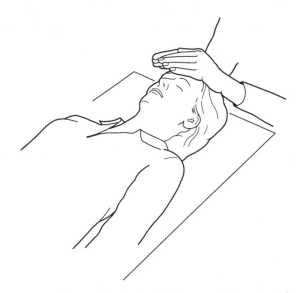

I always suggest to my students that they not place their fingers on the client's face, as some people find this a little claustrophobic, but if the fingers are just curved gently toward the face, as in this illustration, people rarely object to it.

4. These will usually be followed by a hand position next to the ears or on the temples.

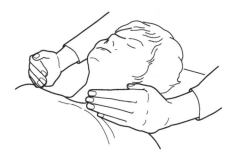

All of the above hand positions allow the Reiki to flow into the head, to treat the brain, nervous system and endocrine system, especially the pineal and pituitary glands, as well as the eyes, ears, nose, sinuses, jaw, mouth, teeth and gums.

5. The next position is on each side of the neck, usually with the practitioner's hands at least 10 centimeters (4 inches) away from the throat, so the client doesn't feel threatened. Never be afraid to tell the practitioner if you want them to move their hands further away in any hand position.

This position treats the throat, tonsils, adenoids and vocal cords, plus the thyroid and parathyroid glands, which control metabolism and growth.

HAND POSITIONS FOR THE FRONT OF THE BODY

1. The first position on the body is the upper chest, but the practitioner will be aware that they need to avoid touching the breasts, so the position of the hands may need to be adjusted depending upon whether the client is male or female, or whether a woman is high or low breasted.

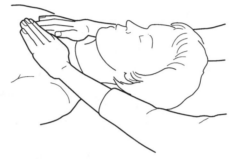

Reiki in this hand position is treating the heart and the whole cardio-vascular system, plus the lymphatic system, the immune system, the lungs and respiratory system, and the thymus gland. The Reiki will also flow from here into the arms and hands.

2. This is followed by a hand position underneath the breasts, on your midriff, the solar plexus.

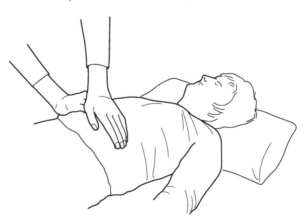

Here Reiki flows into the liver, spleen, pancreas, gallbladder, stomach and the whole of the digestive system.

3. From there, the practitioner's hands will move down to a point on or a fraction below your waist—roughly where your navel is.

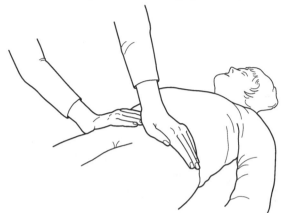

Here Reiki flows into the kidneys and adrenal glands, the lower digestive organs, the prostate, bladder and urinary tract, and parts of the female reproductive system—the uterus, ovaries and Fallopian tubes.

4. The practitioner's hands will then move down to the pelvic area, and different hand positions may be used depending upon whether the client is male or female. The hand position on a female is usually a V shape, as in this illustration, but care is taken to ensure that it does not feel intrusive, so the hands may be moved upward or outward, depending upon the size and shape of the woman client.

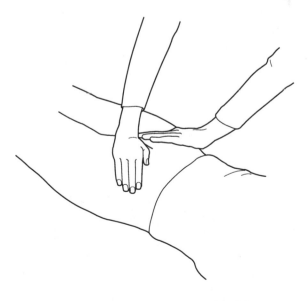

When treating a man, the practitioner will take care not to touch the genital area, so the hands are usually placed on either hip bone, as shown below.

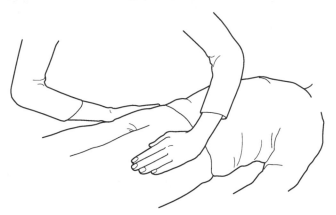

This position treats the bladder, bowels and elimination system, the genitals and the male reproductive organs (testes), as well as again treating the female reproductive organs. In addition, from this position Reiki is believed to treat the whole of the body's structure, including the skeleton, muscles, skin and blood, as well as flowing particularly into the pelvis, hips, legs and feet.

Once the front of the body has been treated, the practitioner may begin to treat your legs and feet (see page 81).

HAND POSITIONS FOR THE BACK OF THE BODY

Once the front of the body has been treated you will often be gently encouraged to turn over to lie on your front so that your back can be treated. Although all the hand positions on the front of the body enable Reiki to flow around the whole body, and therefore into the back as well, treating the back separately allows Reiki to flow even more effectively into some particular parts. The spine, for example, is a very important part of our skeleton, and the four hand positions on the back treat the whole of the spine from the base of the neck down to the coccyx, as well as treating other vital areas again, such as the lungs, heart, liver and kidneys.

1. The first position on the back is usually the shoulders, and from here the Reiki can flow not only into the shoulders and upper back, but also down the arms and into the hands. The practitioner might choose to stand behind your head or beside you for this position.

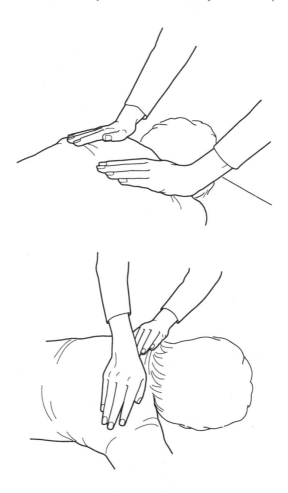

Physically the shoulders are where most of us hold a lot of tension and stress, and this can cause general aches and pains, including headaches, so this hand position treats the muscles and joints in the shoulders, as well as the upper back and the bones, cartilage and nerves in the upper spine.

2. The practitioner will then move their hands down to a position roughly midway between your shoulders and waist, primarily treating the muscles in the upper portion of your back, as well as your spine, heart and lungs.

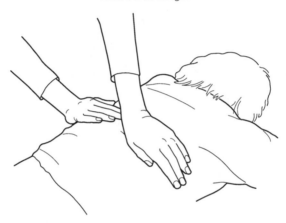

3. The practitioner's hands will move down to your waist area (sometimes just above or just below it), which treats the middle portion of the spine, and allows Reiki to flow again into some important organs such as the pancreas, digestive system, liver, kidneys, spleen and adrenal glands.

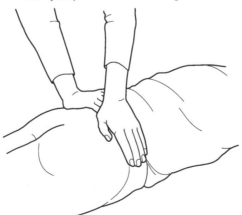

4. The final hand position on the back (unless the legs and feet are treated) is the buttocks, and although some people may find this just a little intrusive, if they are warned about it first they usually don't object.

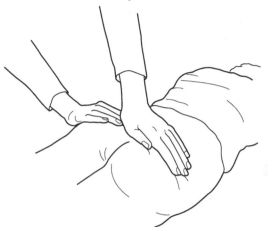

This hand position covers the lower portion of the spine, including the coccyx, and therefore the skeleton, skin, blood and elimination system, as well as the male and female reproductive organs, the genitals, hips, legs and feet.

TREATING THE LEGS AND FEET

As mentioned earlier, some practitioners treat the legs and feet as well as the head and body, although this seems to have been an addition made by some Reiki Masters, rather than by Hayashi or Takata. However, if you have any physical problems with your legs, knees, ankles or feet, do point this out to the practitioner, as they may well decide to give some extra time to those areas even if they are not a part of their usual treatment program. Also, the feet have energy zones that correspond to all parts of the physical body, so giving Reiki to the ankles, heels, toes, and tops and soles of the feet actually sends the healing again to every organ and system within the body.

The legs and feet can be treated in two main ways—each leg individually as a whole, with one of the practitioner's hands on a hip and the other underneath the foot of the same leg (it doesn't matter which leg is treated first); or both legs at the same time, with one of the practitioner's hands being placed on each thigh, then both the knees, shins, ankles and feet, while you lie on your back, and then again the backs of the thighs, knees, calves, ankles and soles of the feet when you lie on your tummy.

TREATING THE ARMS AND HANDS

Very few practitioners include hand positions for the arms and hands, because the Reiki flows to them when the shoulders and upper chest are being treated, but if you have any physical problems in these areas, do tell your therapist, who can then include them in the treatment, immediately after treating the upper chest, after the shoulders have been treated or even right at the end of the treatment. The arms and hands have to be treated individually, as otherwise the practitioner would have to stretch too far over your body, so the easiest way is to have one of their hands on your shoulder, and the other on the hand of the same arm. Alternatively, the practitioner might decide to treat each area separately, holding one hand first on your upper arm with the other hand on your elbow, then moving one hand to your forearm and the other to your wrist, and finally one hand underneath and one on top of your hand, working first on one side of the body, then the other.

BEING TREATED IN A CHAIR

If you are unable to lie on a massage table, or if there isn't one available for your treatment, you can be treated while sitting on a chair. It is a little easier for the practitioner if you can sit in a straight-backed chair, but the treatment can be carried out even if you are only able to sit in an armchair or a wheelchair. Reiki flows easily through the back of any type of chair, so you don't even need to lean forward, which might be a little uncomfortable if you have to hold that position for a while. Some of the hand positions may be combined and the order may be slightly different, to make it a bit easier for the practitioner, but all areas are covered, and the Reiki still flows around the whole of your body.

AFTER THE TREATMENT

Whichever type of treatment you have received, at the end the practitioner will probably do another energy cleansing by sweeping their hands about 15 centimeters (6 inches) in the air above your body, from your head all the way down to your toes, usually three times. This helps to clear any negative energy that might have been released from your body during the treatment, and also smoothes your energy field, so it feels quite pleasant. They might then do a similar action over their own body to cleanse it, while allowing you a little time to "come round" after being so deeply relaxed. If you are having difficulty waking up, they might also gently massage your feet, which is a good grounding exercise.

When you are ready, they should help you to sit up or get off the massage table, and offer you a glass of water. It is a good idea to drink plenty of water for a few days after a Reiki treatment, to help the body to flush out the toxins that may have been dislodged by the Reiki. Some people feel energized immediately after a treatment, while others feel sleepy and incredibly peaceful, but if you feel at all "spaced out," draw this to the attention of your practitioner, who will be able to carry out some grounding activities before they allow you to leave. This is easily achieved by getting you to sit with your feet flat on the floor while the practitioner places one hand on each of your feet, and they then visualize the Reiki energy flowing out through the soles of your feet into the earth below. It is amazing how quickly people return to feeling normal after this simple exercise. However, if this is not sufficient, then standing up and stamping your feet on the ground for about a minute should do the trick.

The Cross Crawl

Another way of grounding yourself is to do an activity called a Cross Crawl, which helps to balance both sides of the brain. Lift your left knee up and touch it with your right hand, then put your left foot down. Lift your right knee up and touch it with your left hand, then put your right foot down on the ground again. Repeat these actions for at least one minute, at a fairly brisk pace—you should be able to manage about 30 times each side in a minute. If you have any trouble balancing, you can actually do this activity while sitting in a chair.

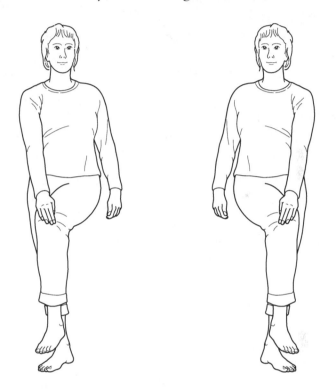

FINDING A REIKI PRACTITIONER

So if you haven't already experienced a Reiki treatment, where can you find a good Reiki practitioner? You may know someone already who does Reiki—a friend, or a member of your own family—so you could approach them. Otherwise, you can contact organizations such as the UK Reiki Federation or the Reiki Association, which have lists of members who work as practitioners either full- or part-time, and there are similar organizations in other parts of the world (see Resources, page 281). There is now a national register of Reiki practitioners in the UK, and you can find details on the websites about the above two organizations as well as about the General Regulatory Council for Complementary Therapies (GRCCT). At present, similar national registers don't exist in other countries, although an Internet search will reveal lists of Masters and Practitioners—see the Resources section for contact details.

Personal recommendation is often the best route, however, and if you ask around it is likely that someone you know has received a treatment, and if they were happy with it, you could contact their practitioner. Alternatively, you could look in local health-food shops, New Age shops, the Yellow Pages, or even your local post office or news dealers, which often have notice boards with business cards or posters put up by local practitioners, or you could approach a holistic health clinic if there are any nearby.

It's a good idea to have an initial chat on the phone first, to gauge whether you feel a practitioner is right for you—and you may have a preference for a male or female practitioner, although as you remain fully clothed during the treatment this is not often a problem. However, don't feel embarrassed if you do prefer a same-sex practitioner—it's just a matter of choice.

Ask how much the practitioners charge—Reiki treatments cost about the same as other complementary therapies such as aromatherapy and reflexology, and last from about 45 minutes to an hour—and perhaps also ask

about their training, and how long they have been practicing. If they are qualified in other therapies they may
have additional skills to offer, if this would be of interest
to you. The best thing is to trust your own judgment.
Because Reiki always works for the greatest and highest
good, you aren't going to be harmed by a Reiki treatment, even if a beginner gives it to you, so be willing to
have a go.

chapter six

THE EFFECTS OF REIKI
AND HOW IT WORKS

Hands-on healing has been used for many thousands of years in virtually every religion, culture and society. Using their own life-force energy (Ki) to heal others is the way some healers work, but they can easily become exhausted if they use too much. Rather like in the case of giving blood too often, the body needs sufficient time to replenish its supply. Some spiritual healers use or help to focus the energies supplied by "unseen friends"— people on the spiritual realm who have agreed to help humanity in this way. Other spiritual healers are able to draw healing energy into themselves, which then flows into the person they are healing.

Reiki healing is similar to this latter form of spiritual healing, although the spiritual healers whom I have attuned to Reiki tell me that the two energies "feel" different as they use them, and that Reiki seems to flow instantaneously, whereas the other healing energy they use builds up more slowly. I do think there are various strands of healing energy which come from the same source, but which perhaps have different vibrationary frequencies and special purposes. Indeed, in the Chinese healing tradition there is a 4,000-year-old text called *The Yellow Emperor's Classic of Internal Medicine*, which states that there are 32 different kinds of Ki!

Reiki can be a valuable and powerful tool to use in the healing process, and one of its advantages is that it does not deplete the energies of the person using it—as I explain in Part 3, a person can become "attuned" to the Reiki energy, and channel it through themselves either for their own healing, or for healing others, so there is no need to use their own precious Ki.

WHAT DOES REIKI DO?

Our whole energy body is responsive to thoughts and feelings, and the flow of Ki becomes disrupted or blocked whenever we consciously or unconsciously accept negative thoughts or feelings about ourselves. Reiki helps to break through these blockages, flowing through the affected part of the energy body—whether that is the aura, the chakras, the meridians or the physical body—charging it with positive energy and raising the vibratory level of the whole energy field. It clears, balances and straightens the energy pathways (i.e., the chakras and meridians) and allows the life force to flow in a healthy and natural way around the whole body. This accelerates the body's natural ability to heal physical ailments, and opens the mind, emotions and spirit to the causes of dis-ease and pain, allowing this knowledge to float to the surface of the mind to promote understanding of the "message" the body's dysfunction is trying to communicate.

THE NEED FOR A CHANGE IN CONSCIOUSNESS

So perhaps we should look at how a change in consciousness—i.e., a change in the ways we think and behave—can help to make healing truly effective and long-lasting. Whether we take a conventional or a metaphysical view, any illness, pain or disease is a signal from the body to indicate that something is wrong. From the conventional viewpoint the indications are fairly basic. If we have a pain in the stomach area then a doctor will look for physical reasons, such as an ulcer, a viral infection or maybe even a grumbling appendix, and will prescribe appropriate treatment, which could range from antibiotics to surgery, and we might also be advised to help ourselves by changing our diet.

From the metaphysical point of view, however, the message is seen at the causative level, so a stomach pain might indicate that there is something going on in your life that you are, literally, finding "hard to stomach." Other examples are a skin rash, which can be a symptom of irritation, or might mean that you are suppressing your normal reactions to something; a bad back could mean that there are problems with the support structure in your life—anything from emotional support (upper back) to money issues (lower back); throat problems could mean you have swallowed your anger and hurt and aren't really expressing what you feel.

Reiki will often alleviate such physical symptoms quite quickly, and because it also works at the causative level, it will help to raise to the surface the issues that are at the root of the physical problem. The trouble is, once the illness or pain has gone away people tend to forget about it, so the underlying message is ignored. No effort is made to look at their lives or to make any necessary changes. In a similar way, many people go to the doctor expecting some pills that will effect an immediate cure without them doing anything about their lifestyle, which may be contributing to their ill health.

For instance, perhaps what you cannot "stomach" is the way you are being treated by your boss or colleagues at work, but once the stomachache goes away you go back to work and carry on as normal. In this case, the cause hasn't been removed, even though the symptom has been relieved. Soon the tension returns, and the stomachache comes back, or is replaced by some other, often more serious, symptom of stress. What is needed in this situation is a change of consciousness, a realization that something must be done about the situation at work.

The problem needs to be tackled in a proactive way. This might mean being assertive and telling your work colleagues that you don't find their attitude acceptable, or talking to your boss about your dissatisfaction. It may even mean that you really need to look for another job which you would find more enjoyable and perhaps better suited to your skills and talents, because sometimes illness can be a "wake-up" call to show us that we're not on the right track.

The main theme here is being involved in your own healing; in taking responsibility for your own health and well-being. We all know that a healthy lifestyle will give us the best possible chance of a healthy body, but most of us are very good at ignoring this fact. But it isn't quite as simplistic as that, because humans are complex, and the causative levels of disease are multileveled. (For more information on the causative factors of illnesses, see Further Reading, page 287.)

REIKI IS SOUL ENERGY

Bringing more spiritual energy (i.e., more of your own soul or spirit) into yourself is what you do when you channel Reiki into or through yourself. Reiki (spiritual energy) is part of your Soul energy, or Higher Self, which is of an even higher and finer vibration than your aura, and it is absolutely pure, loving, wise and totally unaffected by whatever you think, say or do, because it is always directly linked to the Source—or God, or the universe, or whatever term you are happy with. However, the idea that there is more of you than can fit inside your physical body can be quite difficult for some people, although I have already described the fact that your aura can stretch out to 20 meters (66 feet) or more around you, which may be amazing enough. However, your Soul energy is limitless in size, because it is connected to all other Souls, and to the Source/God, at all times, and throughout time. (It is where your life-force energy, or spirit, returns when your physical body dies.) It is vast, infinite and eternal. Hopefully the illustration on page 93 will give you some idea of what I'm talking about.

I've described it in that way to let you see the enormous power and the vast potential of what you have when you access Reiki, because what you are doing is drawing into yourself more of your own spiritual energy— your Soul energy or Higher Self—only a small amount

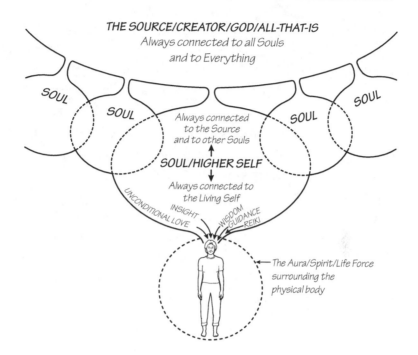

THE SOURCE/CREATOR/GOD/ALL-THAT-IS
*Always connected to all Souls
and to Everything*

SOUL

SOUL

SOUL

SOUL

*Always connected
to the Source
and to other Souls*

SOUL/HIGHER SELF

*Always connected to
the Living Self*

INSIGHT

UNCONDITIONAL LOVE

WISDOM

GUIDANCE

REIKI

*The Aura/Spirit/Life Force
surrounding the
physical body*

of which normally resides within your physical body and aura (i.e., your personal life-force energy, or spirit). The more you use Reiki, and the more often you draw Reiki into yourself for treatments or during meditation, the more of your Higher Self remains within your auric field, which is what raises your energy vibrations. The very high vibrations of your Soul/Higher Self help you to become increasingly "enlightened," that is, energetically lighter than the normally dense physical matter of your body, and this leads to greater spiritual awareness, and to an increasing need for personal growth and spiritual development.

THE WAY REIKI WORKS

1. Healing Practice

Most people are attracted to the healing practice of Reiki in the first place, and usually they think of this as mainly physical healing. Reiki as a healing practice is a hands-on healing technique where spiritual energy (Reiki) is channeled through the hands of the practitioner firstly for self-treatment, and then for treatment of other people, animals and plants. However, because Reiki works holistically, it helps to break through the mental and emotional blocks that have been created by events in people's lives, and heals these on a deep level. The Reiki therefore starts a holistic healing process which can be on any level within the whole person—body, mind, emotions or spirit—but which helps to move that person toward wholeness, health and well-being.

2. Personal Growth

When Reiki flows through a person on a regular basis, deeper levels of blockage are brought to the surface to be healed and then released. In this way the Reiki begins to stimulate personal growth and development. Because Reiki is guided by a higher intelligence, this process always works at a pace that is suited to the individual, so there are no time limits and the effects will be different for each person. As the Reiki slowly breaks down the blockages and barriers that have been created in the mental, emotional and spiritual bodies, it begins a process that enables individuals to become more self-aware, more understanding of themselves and more forgiving of themselves. This in turn leads to a greater acceptance of their true self, which eventually leads to self-love.

3. Spiritual Development

The healing practice and personal growth aspects of Reiki lead to a deepening of our spiritual awareness, the realization of our relationship to All That Is (or God, the Source, the Creator or any other preferred term for a Higher Consciousness). This feeling of connectedness to every living thing brings with it a sense of responsibility, a reverence for all life that is the foundation for a personal view of spirituality and a sense of the sacred within yourself. The very act of treating yourself every day with Reiki is itself a spiritual discipline; the meditative quality of self-treatment encourages a sense of peace and tranquility, and a feeling of oneness with everything around you. It also helps you to recognize more keenly your responsibility for your own health and well-being, so that you can bring about any changes in your life or lifestyle which will enhance your health.

4. Mystic Order

Healing practice, personal growth and spiritual development bring with them further knowledge and experience of Reiki, which in turn brings increased development of insight and an even deeper acceptance of our connection to all consciousness, to the mystery of life. We are so used to wanting to be in control of our lives, to plan, to deliberate, that to surrender to the practice of Reiki, to the inexplicable but often wonderful changes that this energy creates in our lives, can be quite a challenge. But with Reiki running through our lives we can pause to wonder, to appreciate the magical nature of healing which needs no conscious direction, no personal control. There is a mystical beauty in the form of the attunements, and in the often amazing spiritual experiences that students go through during the attunement procedure (see Chapter 8).

When mystery and wonder are inherent in our everyday lives, those lives are richer, and this is the legacy of Reiki. It allows us to accept the unexplainable, to trust the indefinable, and to recognize that if life *is* a mystery, that's all right. We don't have to understand it all. We just have to *be*. Mystic Order is about getting into a space of oneness, of communion with everything in the universe, and you may find this feeling increases as your experience with Reiki increases, until this, too, becomes an essential part of your everyday life.

THE EFFECTS OF REIKI

Because of its power and versatility, Reiki can transform your life in many powerful and wonderful ways. It heals, harmonizes and balances on the four levels of existence, and adjusts itself to the recipient so that each person receives exactly what they need:

◆ **Physical** Reiki supports and accelerates your body's own natural ability to heal itself, helping to alleviate pain and relieve other symptoms while cleansing the body of poisons and toxins. Reiki balances and harmonizes the whole energy body, promoting a sense of wholeness, a state of positive wellness and an overall feeling of well-being. It also helps you to develop a greater awareness of your body's real needs, in relation to such things as nutrition and exercise.

◆ **Emotional** Reiki encourages you to examine your emotional responses, allowing you to let go of negative emotions and promoting the qualities of loving, caring, sharing, trusting and goodwill. It also helps you to channel emotional energy into creativity.

◆ **Mental** Reiki leads to a state of deep relaxation, with the consequent release of stress and tension. It allows you to let go of negative thoughts, concepts and attitudes, replacing them with positivity, peace and serenity. It also enhances your intuitive abilities and encourages you to pursue your personal potential through greater insight and self-awareness.

◆ **Spiritual** Reiki helps you to accept and love your whole self, and fosters a nonjudgmental approach to humankind, allowing you to accept every person not just as a human being, but also as an infinite and eternal soul on a journey of discovery. It promotes the qualities of love, compassion, understanding and acceptance, and encourages you on your personal path toward spiritual development and connectedness with the divine.

WHAT CAN REIKI DO?

Potentially, just about anything! Most people who go for a Reiki treatment want help with a specific physical problem, from frequent headaches or a frozen shoulder, to more serious complaints, although some simply want to be able to relax and cope better with the stresses of modern life. The potential of Reiki is unlimited, so anything can be treated, but it is important to rid yourself of specific expectations of what it will do, and how fast it will perform. Many physical symptoms can be eased very quickly, while others may need a lot of Reiki before starting to respond, but it is essential to remember that it is *your own body* that is actually doing the healing.

Some people report amazing, even miraculous, effects from Reiki treatments, but as mentioned in Chapter 4, "healing" is not *always* the same as "curing," although we unfortunately tend to use the words interchangeably, which creates misunderstanding. Healing doesn't always occur on the physical level first. Because Reiki works holistically, it may be that healing needs to happen first at the emotional level, with the releasing of anger, guilt or hatred, or it may be required first at the mental level, releasing negative thoughts, concepts or attitudes, or at the spiritual level, developing self-awareness, self-understanding and self-love, before the physical symptoms can be addressed.

Just be open-minded, and if you are willing to receive the Reiki (belief in it is not a prerequisite) healing *will* take place, although it might not always be in quite the way you expect, and ultimately if you want the healing to be permanent you have to take responsibility for healing the cause. This may mean changing how you think or the way you relate to other people, or even altering your whole lifestyle, from your diet and home environment to your close relationships, job or career. Surprisingly, perhaps, Reiki can help with these adjustments too, allowing you to approach the changes in a relaxed way.

Because Reiki is guided by a Higher Intelligence, it always finds its way to those areas of the physical body and/or the energy body most in need of healing, without any conscious direction from either the healer or the person being healed, and it adjusts to suit the recipient, so that each person receives as much or as little healing as they need at that particular time.

In Chapter 5, I outlined what would be treated physically by each hand position. Now I introduce some of the metaphysical effects that could be attributed to each hand position. Clearly the exact effects will depend upon each individual person and their needs, but this will give you some idea of what areas of your life might be treated.

Crown	Encourages inner knowledge and awareness, spirituality, a sense of unity and connectedness to everyone and everything, and feelings of fulfillment, completion and enlightenment.
Eyes	Encourages intuition, insight and imagination, sometimes promoting the development of inner vision, clairvoyance or other psychic gifts.
Ears	The willingness to listen to higher guidance, and the possible development of clairaudient skills. This position also works to promote healthy sleep patterns.
Back of the Head	Because this works on the visual cortex it also encourages inner vision, often activating the imagination and stimulating visualization. However, it also helps to promote restful sleep.

Throat
Encourages the ability to communicate honestly and effectively, and promotes creativity and self-expression, including expression through music and the voice.

Heart
Encourages unconditional love and good relationships, empathy, kindness and compassion toward others and oneself, self-acceptance and understanding, and a willingness to both give and receive.

Solar Plexus
Helps you to develop willpower, self-control, recognition of your need for personal authority and autonomy, self-esteem and self-determination, as well as an understanding of your potential and your purpose in life, and encourages an increase in your overall energy.

Navel Area
Has an effect on an individual's sexuality, emotions and romantic relationships, aspects of intimacy and sharing, and all facets of sensuality, including the appetite for food, sex and other pleasures. In addition, it encourages creativity in all its forms, and an appreciation of all the senses.

Pelvic Area
Feelings about your physical body, as well as your feelings of security and trust and sense of survival, which also covers issues about money, home, work, and your sense of belonging and interaction with nature and the earth.

Shoulders	Shoulders are where we carry responsibility, often "shouldering" other people's burdens, and where we hold on to the stress of not doing what we want to do.
Mid-Back	This section of the back is linked with feeling emotionally unsupported, unloved or misunderstood, and the heart is naturally linked to love and joy, while the lungs are connected to deep-seated issues about our capacity for, or fear of, life itself.
Waist	This is where our bodies bend physically, so metaphysically this area can show whether we are rigid and resentful, or flexible and accepting in our attitudes, whether we can adequately balance our own needs with others' demands.
Buttocks	This is where we can "sit on" our feelings, especially fears of lack, whether that is materially or emotionally, and there are parental issues linked with this, as we tend to internalize our parents' expectations. Sometimes we can develop extra weight in this area, as another way of smothering our real feelings or hiding our fears.
Legs and Feet	Our legs and feet connect us with the ground, carry us and move us forward in life, enabling us to walk, run, skip or climb, as well as to stand still, so problems here often relate to resistance or reluctance to move in a particular direction, or a fear of the future.

| **Arms and Hands** | Our arms enable us to interact physically with people and things. They can indicate how much effort we put into life, how we express ourselves and how we embrace life itself. Hands can be literally how we "handle" life. |

Because Reiki always flows to the areas of the physical body or energy bodies that need it, and because the classic 12 hand positions enable the Reiki to flow easily and effectively into all the major chakra points, other hand positions are not really necessary, although as mentioned in Chapter 5, if your practitioner uses additional hand positions, or different ones from those I have described, that is fine—there is room for some individuality in the practice of Reiki.

You should now have some understanding of the healing process and an idea of what it is like to experience a Reiki treatment, and should know about the effects of Reiki and how it works. In Part 3 I describe how you can learn to do Reiki yourself, explain what an attunement is and discuss how Reiki training has developed over time in the West.

part three

LEARNING REIKI

chapter seven

THE LEVELS OF TRAINING

Reiki is probably the simplest and easiest holistic healing method available to us, so anyone can learn to use it, whatever their age or gender, religion or origin (except perhaps for very young children, who would not understand its significance). "Learning" Reiki is really a misnomer, as I explain fully in Chapter 8, because the ability to let this healing energy flow through you is passed on from the Reiki Master to the student in a sacred ceremony called the attunement or initiation. As soon as you have been attuned you have Reiki and can use it. You therefore don't need any specific knowledge or experience—just a willingness to let this healing energy flow through you, and a little time to attend a Reiki course—most first-level courses are held over just a day or two. From the time you receive your first Reiki attunement, you are able to call upon this spiritual energy at any time, in any place, for as long as you live. The ability to channel Reiki doesn't wear off or wear out, so even if you don't use it for years, Reiki is still available to you, although you may need to practice a little to reestablish the same quantity of flow.

It is wonderful to be able to develop the ability to heal so quickly, yet so permanently. Your first Reiki attunement reactivates a pure channel for the healing energy that flows from the crown chakra through to the heart chakra, and then to the hands (see the illustration, page 136). Some people report "seeing" the Reiki energy as a vortex of universal life-force energy pouring into the crown chakra of the practitioner, and then out of each hand. The Reiki flows through this pure channel, but it is important to note that when you are treating someone or something else, it is *pulled* by the recipient, not *pushed* by you. It is not possible to *force* healing into anyone, and this all takes place at the subconscious level, so if you are treating a person, they do not need to "think" the Reiki in, or mentally say "let Reiki flow into me" over and over again. And neither do you—all you need, once you have been attuned, is to *intend* that the Reiki flows, and it will begin to flow, provided the person or animal needs it on some level (physical, mental, emotional or spiritual).

REIKI LEVELS OF TRAINING

Reiki is taught by qualified Reiki Masters (teachers), and there are three levels, sometimes referred to as "degrees" (e.g., Reiki First Degree, Reiki Second Degree)—although this does not refer to any academic level or qualification. One of the definitions of the word "degree" is "a stage in intensity or amount" (*Concise Oxford English Dictionary*), so it is another way of referring to the level of training or the amount of Reiki that can be accessed.

At each level of attunement (Reiki 1, 2 or 3) the vibra-tionary rate of your energy field is heightened and you are able to tap into a higher, wider channel of Reiki. Then whenever you intend to use Reiki, simply thinking about it, or holding your hands out in readiness to use it, will activate it. The Reiki will be drawn in through your crown chakra, then it flows down the Reiki channel, through the brow, throat and heart chakras, and then down each arm, eventually streaming out of the palm chakras. As you use Reiki in this way, the majority of the flow will come out of your hands, to be used either on yourself in a self-treatment, or for other people, animals, plants, and so on. However, some Reiki will flow out of the heart chakra into your own energy body, and from there will flow gently around your energy system. This is one of the reasons why a Reiki practitioner feels so good after carrying out a treatment on another person—they have also been receiving some Reiki.

Each Reiki Master may have a slightly different way of training people, and I explain more in Chapter 9 about the changes that have happened within the Western and Eastern ways of Reiki training. However, the basics of at least one attunement and some brief instruction on how to use Reiki will usually be included.

Reiki First Degree/Reiki 1

This is the basic course for everyone, from people who mainly wish to use Reiki on themselves, their friends and family—and perhaps their pets and plants—to those who wish to go on to become Reiki practitioners. It is usually held over at least one day, often two days, or sometimes over four evenings (normally a minimum of 12 hours' teaching), and some Masters offer a free introductory talk sometime before the course, so that you can find out more about it, have a chance to experience receiving a short informal Reiki treatment for yourself, and be sure that the course is right for you.

Traditional Reiki First Degree courses include four attunements, and should also cover a comprehensive explanation of the Usui system of Reiki natural healing, including the story of how it was rediscovered by Dr. Usui. Full training should be given in the basic form of treatment—hand positions on the head and body for treating yourself and others, and advice on how to give treatments for injuries or accidents, as well as explanations of how to use Reiki with animals and plants. Plenty of time should be allowed for practicing on yourself and on other students under the supervision of the Reiki Master, and you should be encouraged to ask questions and share your experiences during the course.

The above description refers to the traditional teaching of Usui Reiki, normally held over at least two days, but there are variations. For example, some Masters use the Usui/Tibetan system taught originally by the American Reiki Master William Lee Rand, where it is usual to carry out only one integrated attunement (although it is possible to use four attunements with this system, too) and the course is normally held over only one day. This works perfectly well, although while the traditional method allows the energy to build up slowly and gently over several sessions, in the single-attunement method the energy is "delivered" all at once.

The four-attunement method is probably closer to the original Japanese way of training, and bearing in mind that the purpose of the attunements is to "bring you into harmony" with the energy, each attunement seems to work at a different level:

Attunement 1	Your emotions and heart chakra.
Attunement 2	Your communications and throat chakra.
Attunement 3	Your intuition and the brow or third eye chakra.
Attunement 4	Your spiritual level, and the crown chakra, permanently connecting you with spiritual consciousness and sealing the Reiki channel open, so that you always have access to it.

However, after many years of carrying out such attunements, I can now psychically "see" what is happening inside each person's energy field, and something also occurs at another level in reverse order. The light of Reiki "locks into" first the crown chakra, then the brow chakra, followed by the throat chakra and finally the heart chakra, from where it gently spreads around the whole energy field, tinting it with violet light—a beautiful "sight," and one which confirms to me that the student is filled with Reiki and the attunement is complete.

The hand positions for treatment may also vary slightly from one Master to another, depending upon how they were taught, and many Masters teach additional hand positions for the legs and feet, or for specific purposes. Other variations can include meditations, energy cleansing, chanting, group treatments, aura and chakra work, or a Master may choose to place particular emphasis on treating animals or working on healing the environment.

Reiki Second Degree/Reiki 2

This course is only available to those who have already completed First Degree, who want to deepen their understanding of Reiki and its uses. It is recommended for people who wish to become Reiki practitioners, and for those who want to use Reiki more effectively on their own inner development. Some Reiki Masters ask that you leave at least three months between Reiki 1 and Reiki 2, to allow your own energies to effectively assimilate the higher vibrations of the Reiki, while others suggest only three weeks between, or allow you to progress to Second Degree the day after taking the First Degree course, so you take Reiki 1 and Reiki 2 in a single weekend.

However, the traditional Usui Reiki 2 course normally takes two days (or four sessions), and includes at least one, sometimes two, energy attunements which intensify your inner healing channel—I believe to as much as four times that received with First Degree—and which many people find to be a very profound experience. When I "see" what is happening inside a person's energy field when they are experiencing a traditional Usui Second Degree attunement, I see the Reiki flowing through the crown, brow, throat and heart chakras, which have already been attuned, and then see the light of Reiki "lock into" the solar plexus and sacral chakras, after which it dissipates around their whole auric field.

During a Reiki 2 course you are taught three sacred symbols, together with sacred mantras (sounds from

Sanskrit or Japanese) which are used alongside them. The symbols are calligraphic shapes that are drawn in the air with the hand, or they can be drawn in the imagination if other people might see them being drawn physically, as it is traditional not to disclose them to anyone who has not done Reiki 2—which is why the actual shapes are not reproduced in this book.

1. **The Power (or Focus) Symbol**
    This symbol is probably the most versatile of the three given at Second Degree. It can be used alone (it is the only symbol which can be used by itself), or in combination with either or both of the other two symbols. There are many possible uses for the power symbol, but its main features are for empowering, cleansing and protecting, as well as for use in general healing.

2. **The Harmony (Mental/Emotional) Symbol**
    This symbol's main functions are to help to restore psychological and emotional balance, to raise sensitivity and receptivity, and to bring peace and harmony.

3. **The Distant (Connection) Symbol**
    Using this symbol cuts through, or goes beyond, time and space, bringing all time into the Now, and all space into the Here. The best analogy I can come up with is that the Distant Symbol is an energetic equivalent of a time machine, because it enables you to connect with anything, anywhere, at any time, so it allows you to "send" healing to anyone in any location, whether that is the next room or another country, and at any time, including the present, the past and the future.

You are also taught some specific techniques which use one or more of the symbols, such as distant (absent) healing, methods to intensify the energy flow in "hands-on" treatments, how to heal life situations or deep-seated emotional or psychological problems, as well as how to use Reiki to heal the planet, or for your own further personal and spiritual development.

Some Masters include a number of traditional Japanese techniques, plus additional topics, such as cleansing the aura with special herbs (called a "smudge" mix), developing sensitivity in your hands to enable you to scan the aura for energy variations, meditations to meet Reiki guides, empowering affirmations and goals with Reiki, cleansing crystals or spaces using Reiki, or many other aspects of Reiki which become possible at Second Degree level. Most of these are not strictly necessary, and some, like using crystals, are not really a part of Reiki training at all, but they can often enhance the experience for students and show them just part of the immense potential of Reiki at this level. Occasionally some Reiki Masters put on extra one- or two-day courses specially for students who have already had some experience of using the Second Degree symbols, to enable them to acquire these and other additional techniques.

Practice time should be available on the Reiki 2 course for any of the techniques taught, especially those that involve treating people, but participants should expect to put aside time over the following few months to practice both hands-on and distant treatments, and many Masters will not issue a Second Degree certificate until this extra practice has been done, and may expect a case-study journal to be submitted. There should, of course, be plenty of time allowed to ask questions and share experiences.

Reiki Third Degree/Reiki 3/Reiki Master

This is the level of a Reiki Master, and is for those who have already practiced at Second Degree Level for several years, and feel drawn to demonstrate their commitment to Reiki by learning more advanced techniques and becoming Masters/teachers. The traditional training is extensive, usually taking a year or more working individually with a Master learning and practicing all aspects of Reiki. However, most Masters now teach this level as a short course, which can range from one, two or three days, up to a week or more. Also, some Masters allow their students to progress to Reiki 3 quite quickly—within a few weeks or months—whereas others insist on a minimum of two or three years' experience of Reiki beforehand.

Traditionally this level includes the Usui Master symbol (see page 115), and another attunement that enhances the ability to channel Reiki, possibly up to ten times that at Reiki Second Degree. However, the Usui/Tibetan system, which is the one now most commonly taught in the West, includes another two symbols in addition to the Usui Master symbol, and it is often split into two parts, sometimes known as Reiki 3A, or Advanced Reiki Training, or Reiki Master Practitioner, and this is then followed at a later date by Reiki Master Teacher, so this will include two attunements, one at each level.

The Reiki Master student should be taught and have time to practice the attunement process for each level, and should also have the opportunity to learn how to organize Reiki classes and to practice teaching First and Second Degree classes under the supervision of the Master. There needs also to be some work between Master and student on personal and spiritual growth, so that the student fully understands the commitment that the role of Reiki Master requires. It is often expected that a Master will teach only the first two levels of Reiki for at least two or three years in order to gain the considerable experience necessary to teach someone else the Master level, although some Masters don't insist on this.

It is really important to realize the distinction between the Master level and the other two levels. Becoming a Reiki Master is not simply gaining another qualification. It is actually committing yourself to the mastery of Reiki, which is a lifelong task. At Master level, working on your spiritual development is no longer optional—it is essential—and this inevitably engenders considerable changes. These changes could be in your diet, lifestyle, job, minor or major relationships, where you live, or any other aspect of your life, as well as in you personally. If you really like the life you're living now, and don't want any parts of it to change, then perhaps it isn't the right time to become a Reiki Master!

Remember that Reiki is a spiritual discipline, but unlike most other spiritual disciplines, it does not take years of study and dedication before you are granted access to it. Anyone can take Reiki, at least at the first level, regardless of their age, gender, nationality, spiritual background or beliefs.

The Reiki Master/Empowerment Symbol

Use of the Usui Master symbol in conjunction with Reiki creates a much stronger channel between the physical self and the Higher Self, allowing you to access divine wisdom and insight more easily. All the qualities of Reiki, including the actions of the other symbols, are enhanced when you use the Usui Master symbol. One of its main uses is during the attunements, or spiritual empowerments, but it can also be used when giving Reiki treatments or to empower any other kind of healing, including manifesting or personal transformation work.

PREPARING FOR A REIKI COURSE

When you choose to take Reiki, at any level, it means you have reached an important point on your life path, and are acknowledging that stage of your development. A Reiki attunement is a very special experience, as I have already mentioned, because Reiki is not simply a healing technique; it is an important tool for personal and spiritual growth. The experience can be enhanced if you can bring your physical, mental, emotional and spiritual bodies into harmony and balance over three to seven days before a course commences. There are some aspects of our normal, busy lifestyles that are not particularly conducive to this balance, so the following suggestions are optional. (In respect of the dietary advice, check with your doctor if you have any reason to suspect that a change of diet could be detrimental to you.)

- Many people find it very helpful to go on a gentle "detox" diet for a few days before an attunement. This basically means eating only fresh raw vegetables and fruit (preferably organic) and drinking only water.
- If you are used to fasting, you might wish to start with 24 hours on a water or fruit/vegetable juice fast.
- If that all sounds a bit too drastic, then even if you are not a vegetarian, you may find it helpful to cut out meat and fish for a few days before the course, substituting lots of fresh vegetables and fruit, as this helps to cleanse your physical system. (Meat and fish may contain small quantities of drugs or other toxins.) Cutting down on (or eliminating) processed and packaged foods is helpful, too, as most contain preservatives or additives.
- It is extremely beneficial to drink plenty of water (still, not carbonated). Six to eight glasses a day (about 2 liters) is recommended. (If you have any problems with water retention, or other health problems where taking in more liquids could be detrimental, check this with your doctor first.)
- Cut out alcohol for a few days before and after the attunements, and during the Reiki course itself, and try to minimize your consumption of caffeine drinks, sweets and chocolate during that time.
- If you smoke, try to cut down for several days beforehand, and smoke as little as possible during and immediately after the course.
- Try to reduce or eliminate altogether the time you spend in any activities or situations that carry negative energy (this includes watching TV news, or violent or fear-inducing TV programs; listening to loud music; reading newspapers).

- Actively release any negative emotions such as anger, fear, jealousy or hatred by imagining them in a bubble of light that you allow to float up to the universe to be healed. Then imagine yourself in a bubble of light as a sacred space.
- Try to spend some time quietly in meditation, or taking quiet walks in the countryside, as these are useful activities to "de-stress" you, so that you will be more in tune with the nature of the course.

For the course itself, you will probably find it best to wear comfortable, loose clothing—tracksuits, leggings, T-shirts, sweatshirts or similar are ideal, as they don't have tight waistbands. Wearing layers is helpful, too, as some people find they get very hot when the Reiki energy is flowing through them, and cool when they are just sitting quietly. Some Masters provide a manual or course notes, but you will almost certainly find it useful to take along a notebook and pen.

ACTIVITY—VISUALIZATION TO PREPARE FOR A REIKI COURSE

- One of the ways recommended to prepare for a Reiki course is to let go of negative emotions, and this visualization helps you to do this. (Of course, preparing for a Reiki course isn't the only beneficial time for letting go of negative emotions, so do try this visualization even if you're not about to undertake Reiki training.) Before you begin, you will need to be in a comfortable, quiet place where you won't be disturbed, and it would be helpful to go through the relaxation stage of the visualization on page 57 (clearing your aura) before starting this particular guided imagery—so start with the introductory sequence of relaxing all parts of the body.

◆ Begin by imagining that you are standing on a path in sunlit woodland at the foot of a beautiful mountain. Use all your senses to connect with this image. Look down at your feet to see what kind of shoes you are wearing. Look up at the blue sky, and feel the warmth of the sun on your face, and a gentle breeze ruffling your hair. Imagine yourself putting out your hand to touch something—the rough bark of a tree, or the softness of a blade of grass. Smell the pine-scented air.

◆ Then start to walk along the path, seeing or sensing the beautiful trees around you as the path begins to wind upward, and as you are walking, you feel that the path is becoming narrower, and the woodland is becoming thicker and darker, and you suddenly realize that you are carrying a very heavy bag. You stop for a moment, and you take off the bag to examine the contents. You see that this bag is labeled "Fear," and when you look inside you can see or sense images of all the things that make you fearful. You realize that you don't have to carry this heavy burden of fear around with you any longer. You can choose to leave this heavy bag here beside the woodland path, and move on, knowing that if you really need any of these fears, you can choose to pick up any of them from this bag on your way back down the mountain, should you wish to do so.

◆ Now you stride on up the path, and the trees become thinner and the sun warms you as you climb further, but the path is becoming steeper, and you realize that you are carrying other heavy bags on your back. You go a little further and decide that it's time to examine one of the other bags that you have brought along, so you take off the bag that is labeled "Anger" and look inside. You see or sense images of people or situations that frequently trigger angry emotions in you, but as you look at them you realize that you can choose not to react to these triggers anymore. You can leave all your anger in this bag, so you place the bag down and leave it beside the path, because such emotions are no longer appropriate for you on this journey, but you know that you can pick them up later, if you choose to do so.

◆ You continue climbing, and now you are above the trees, and the sun is getting hotter and hotter, and you eagerly take off another bag to look inside it. This bag is labeled "Guilt," and inside it you find images of all the times when you have felt guilty or jealous or resentful or grudging or possessive, but now you realize that you can let go of those feelings, so you put down the bag and leave it beside the path, feeling much lighter as you step out on the path again, although you know that if you wish to, you may pick up any of these feelings again on your way back down the mountain.

◆ Higher and higher you climb, and you are now almost at the top of the mountain, but the way is really steep now, and you have another bag that is becoming very, very heavy. You decide to take it off, and you see that it is labeled "Worry," and inside you can see or sense all the things you worry about, all the thoughts that have kept you awake at night, all the judgments and prejudices and attitudes that have held you back, all tangled together in a great heap. With a feeling of great relief, you realize that you can also leave all your worries bundled up in this bag, and you place the bag beside the path, knowing that if any of these worries are necessary, you can pick them up again on your way back.

◆ Now you just have a little way to go, but the path has become dangerously narrow and so steep that you are having to scramble up the rocks. The last bag on your back has become too cumbersome and heavy to continue with, so you take it off and gratefully put it on the ground. You notice that it is labeled "Hatred," and when you look inside you are surprised to find any images of such a strong emotion, yet in the darkest recesses of your mind there are people and incidents that have triggered this feeling in you, but now you can release this negative emotion by leaving this bag, like the others, beside the path.

◆ You now feel so light that the path is easy, and you find yourself right at the top of the mountain, and as you stand there the streams of sunlight become beautiful beams of rainbow-colored light, and you feel your whole body and energy field suffused with glorious color as each chakra and each layer of your aura is cleansed of negativity, leaving you feeling peaceful, yet refreshed and grateful to be so vibrantly alive.

◆ The rainbow light recedes, and you begin to make your way back down the mountain. As you come to the last bag you left beside the path you realize that you don't need to pick up any negative emotions anymore, and you find that the bag has changed, and instead of "Hatred" the label now says "Love," so you pick up the bag and find that it is as light as a feather. Moving further down the path you come to the next bag, and find that the label "Worry" has been replaced with "Joy," and you pick up the bag and find that it, too, is as light as a feather. Walking quickly now, you reach the next bag and find that the label has changed from "Guilt" to "Freedom," and you swing the bag easily onto your shoulder and move even more quickly down the path. As you reach the next bag you see that the "Anger" label has changed to "Peace," so you eagerly pick up the bag and begin to run down the path. When you reach the very first bag you put down, which had been labeled "Fear," you find the label reads "Trust," and you happily pick up the bag and carry it lightly with the rest.

◆ As you reach the bottom of the mountain where you first began, you look with a new appreciation of the beauty around you—the bright colors, the warm sunlight, the delicious scents in the breeze. You sit down on the grass and spread out the bags you have brought back down the mountain—Love, Joy, Freedom, Peace and Trust. Each is full, yet the bags weigh hardly anything at all, and you realize that you can choose to release any negative emotions, and fill your life with these and other positive emotions and feelings from now on, allowing you to move lightly through life.

◆ Now your awareness slowly begins to return, and you can hear the sounds around you, and become aware of your body again, and you may want to stretch a little, or wriggle your fingers and toes, and then whenever you are ready, you can open your eyes and feel relaxed, yet fully awake and alert.

AFTER THE REIKI COURSE

Some people have a shift in consciousness immediately after a Reiki course, experiencing colors and sounds more intensely, or feeling a buzzing or heightened sensitivity in the crown center or a sense of floating or even slight light-headedness. If this does happen, do accept it as absolutely normal. Any such sensations usually fade after a short time, anyway. Many people find they are very hungry during and after a Reiki course, or that they need much more sleep than usual. Others, conversely, seem to have lots of extra energy. Most people do feel on a "high" when they've finished the course, though, so I would recommend that you slip back into normal life as gently as possible afterward. This may not be easy, as often the courses are held on a weekend and you may have to get back to work on Monday. Even so, if you do have the chance, perhaps you could take the Monday as a day's holiday, and just allow yourself to "come down" slowly, maybe sleeping in and then spending the day doing gentle things like walking in the countryside, reading, meditating or listening to relaxing music—or a bit of each.

21-DAY CLEARING CYCLE

At each level of attunement the vibrationary rate at which you operate is raised, and in order for this to happen there has to be a clearing of old physical, mental, emotional and spiritual patterns and thoughts that inhibit the growth of the consciousness. One of the major effects, therefore, is what is called the 21-day Clearing Cycle, where your whole energy body is cleansed and cleared by the Reiki.

During the first week after a Reiki course, this clearing takes place gradually by proceeding up through the chakras—the root or base chakra on day one, the sacral chakra on day two, and so on up to the crown chakra on day seven. During the second and third weeks this clearing is repeated in the same way—base chakra on day one, sacral chakra on day two, and so on. I usually describe this as a sort of energetic "spring cleaning" where the Reiki gently flows through and begins to break down the blockages in your whole energy system.

As the blocks that are preventing your progress are brought forward, they need to be released by your physical, emotional, mental and spiritual bodies. The effects of this release can vary from feeling more emotional or irritable than usual, or having the urge to laugh or cry, to a sense of detachment and the need to spend more time alone. Sometimes you may experience a temporary "healing crisis," such as a cold, but this is simply a way to release toxins out of the body and is perfectly natural (if a little uncomfortable). However, this does not always happen, so don't turn it into a "self-fulfilling prophecy." Also, it is important to realize that Reiki always works for the highest good, so be completely trusting when you open to the flow of Reiki, and just let it be. Trust Reiki to know what's best and to do it, then know that this is done, and give thanks for the blessings—and wait to see how the healing manifests. You can make the whole process much easier for yourself, however, by following these recommendations:

- It is really important to do a full self-treatment (at least half an hour) every day during this clearing cycle (see Chapter 10 for instructions).
- It is equally important to drink lots of water—at least six to eight glasses (approximately 2 liters) each day. This needs to be pure water (i.e., other drinks like tea or coffee, cordials, fizzy drinks, etc., don't count), but can be either bottled or tap water—still, not sparkling— although you can include drinks such as fruit or herbal teas in your total amount. (If you have any health problems related to water retention, seek medical advice before drinking extra water.)
- You may also find it useful to repeat the Reiki principles to yourself—see Chapter 12.

Over the three weeks you will probably notice a gradual strengthening of the Reiki as you use it, and other changes in yourself, too. For this purpose it is good to keep a journal of your "Reiki journey" for the first few weeks, where you can record what you experience during self-treatment, or during treatments of friends, family, pets or plants. You may also find it a good idea to write down any vivid dreams, emotional episodes, feelings, and meditations you experience, or changes you feel are taking place in yourself, and perhaps link them to the particular chakra that is being "cleared" on that day (see the descriptions in Chapter 4).

CHOOSING A REIKI MASTER

Inevitably there are differences between individual Reiki Masters, regardless of how they were trained. Some are excellent, inspirational teachers, some are fairly average, and a few are not very good at what they do—as in any profession. But you will want to make sure that you find the right Master to train you, whichever level you are wishing to take. Just as I believe Reiki finds you at precisely the right time in your life, rather than you finding it, I believe you always find the right Reiki Master, too. Use your intuition, and recommendations from people you know. Someone with years of experience teaching Reiki is probably (although not always) going to be better at it than someone who has just completed their training. A Reiki Master who previously spent years working as a Reiki practitioner can offer better advice on how to treat clients than one who has only treated family and friends. Being taught individually, or in a class of six to ten people, will allow you to gain more personal attention than being taught in a class for 20, 30, 50 or more.

Allow yourself to be drawn to the right person, which will usually be a Reiki Master whom you feel has integrity, behaves in a caring and supportive manner, and has the kinds of attitudes and beliefs with which you feel comfortable. Don't be afraid to ask them questions, such as:

- How long have they been doing Reiki? (i.e., when did they do Reiki First Degree?)
- How long have they been a Reiki Master, and what is their lineage (see page 129)?
- How long do the classes last, and what is covered in each class?
- How many students are there in a typical class?
- How long do they advise you to wait between each level of training?

- Will the training be in traditional Usui Reiki, or Usui/Tibetan? Do they also teach other forms of Reiki?
- How much do they charge for the training? Why do they charge that amount?
- What support from the Master is available for students after the course is ended?
- Do they have a Reiki sharing group in your area that you could join?
- Will you get a certificate?
- Do they offer an introductory evening where you can find out more about Reiki?
- Do they offer any other supporting training, such as techniques from the Japanese traditions, or classes on how to deal with clients?

Be aware of what issues are most important to you. Do you want someone with a very spiritual approach, or would you prefer someone very practical and down-to-earth? Are you looking for one-on-one training, or would you prefer to be part of a class? Are you looking for a fairly fast progression, or would you prefer to take your time and practice each level before moving on?

However analytical you are, in the end all you can do is follow your heart, and trust that the experience you have will be the right one for you. You may find it surprising, but when the time is right everything just seems to fall effortlessly into place.

chapter eight

BECOMING ATTUNED
TO REIKI

In Chapter 7 I described the different levels of Reiki training, but what they all have in common is the way in which the flow of Reiki energy is initially acquired, and that is through an attunement. So what is an attunement? This chapter provides an insight into the beauty and power of the ceremonial spiritual empowerment through which you acquire the ability to channel the healing energy we call Reiki.

THE LINEAGE SYSTEM OF KNOWLEDGE TRANSFERENCE IN REIKI

Reiki cannot be "learned" in any of the ways with which we in the West are familiar. It doesn't actually require any *learning*, in the traditional sense, because it is not knowledge based—it is experience based. You cannot acquire the ability to channel Reiki by reading this book, or attending a lecture, or watching a television program, video or DVD, although you can learn how to *use* Reiki in those ways—for instance, where to place your hands when carrying out a Reiki treatment.

The ability to channel Reiki energy is passed on from a teacher (Reiki Master) to a student through a lineage system, which simply means that each Reiki Master can trace their lineage back to the founder of Reiki Ryoho, Mikao Usui, rather like through a family tree. This lineage system is thought to be important because of the manner in which Reiki is passed from Master to student—by means of a spiritual empowerment that we call an "attunement." In Buddhism a spiritual empowerment is a familiar but very special element in spiritual practice, where knowledge, insight and ability are passed from a Sensei (respected teacher) by thought and intention deep into the student's mind, body and spirit, and it usually takes place as part of a sacred ceremony. Dr. Usui experienced a powerful enlightenment experience on Mount Kurama (see page 7), when he received a spiritual empowerment, which gave him a deep knowledge and understanding of the Reiki symbols, and the ability to heal. The spiritual empowerment which is carried out by a Reiki Master today is similar in nature, but less powerful, since Dr. Usui received the whole understanding and the full strength of Reiki in one single empowerment, directly from the Source, which also allowed him to achieve "satori," meaning spiritual enlightenment.

So a Reiki attunement is really an ancient spiritual empowerment, similar in nature to the empowerments given today in Tibetan Buddhism and other spiritual schools, where the teacher transfers energy and existential knowledge to the student through a form of initiation. In Usui Reiki there are a number of these spiritual empowerments spread out between the various levels of training, so that the student has time to "acclimatize" to the levels of energy involved. Within the Reiki community we usually call these sacred ceremonies initiations or attunements, as they "initiate" the student into a new life with Reiki (initiate means "to begin") and "attune" the student to the unique vibrations of the Reiki spiritual healing energy (attune means "to bring into harmony with"). The attunement activates an energetic channel in the student, through which the Reiki energy can flow from the Source, through the student's energy body and out through the hands.

Actually, the attunement is "reopening" or strengthening a preexisting channel to our enlightened selves (our Soul/Spirit/Higher Self), that part of us which is always and completely connected to the Source/God/All That Is. Most people assume and believe that as the Reiki energy enters them through their crown chakra, it must come from outside themselves, from God, the universe or the Source, or whatever term they feel comfortable with. In essence this is true, but I believe we have slightly misinterpreted the way in which we access this divine energy, and it only *seems* external because as humans living in physical bodies we have a limited awareness of our whole existence, and cannot "see" the full extent and potential of our being, our Soul/Spirit/Higher Self, and our eternal connectedness to the divine Source. The "spiritual empowerment" that takes place during the attunement is just that—it empowers a part of our spirit, Reiki—which we didn't consciously know how to access before, so that we become aware of it for the first time, and can begin to use it. (See also Chapter 6, and illustration on page 93.)

Drawing into our physical bodies more energy of a higher energetic vibration from our Soul/Spirit/ Higher Self raises our consciousness and starts a process that continues throughout life—a process of slowly raising awareness of our life purpose, of what we are here to achieve, and how we can achieve it. This is working on a very subtle level, and many people who use Reiki, particularly those who don't use it regularly, are unaware of it. But Reiki works as a catalyst for change, bringing to the surface those aspects of life that are blocking our spiritual progress. Sometimes this can seem a challenging process, but it is always beneficial, as Reiki is divinely guided, and always works for our highest and greatest good.

THE ATTUNEMENT PROCESS

The attunement process makes Reiki unique, and is the reason why the ability to heal can be developed so quickly, yet so permanently. As mentioned (see page 129), the attunement is a sacred ceremony of spiritual empowerment, and the actual process is kept secret until Reiki 3 training is taken to become a Reiki Master, when students are taught the Usui Master symbol (and in many cases two additional symbols from the Usui/Tibetan system developed by William Lee Rand) and the attunement procedure for each of the levels of Reiki.

The attunement forms a connection between the student, the Master and Reiki, and is carried out in what I would describe as "sacred space." When the Reiki Master intentionally "brings in" the energy in preparation for performing the attunement (i.e., accesses and brings in more of their own divine spiritual energy), this has the effect of altering the energetic space around the Master and student(s), filling it with Reiki to provide a protective environment, and also filling the Reiki Master with intense and very tangible Reiki energy.

Reiki Masters differ in the way they arrange things for the attunements, as some prefer to work one to one, while others like to work with groups, but each attunement is usually carried out in silence, with perhaps some soft, relaxing music playing in the background, and each student sits with their eyes closed and their hands held in the "Gassho" or prayer position, palms together in front of the chest. At various stages during the process there may be some gentle touching on the student's head and hands, and they may be asked to raise their hands above their head for a few moments, but everything is very gentle, supportive and restful. The attunement is a very special, meditative experience, and the silent contemplation with eyes closed occurs for two reasons. The first is obviously because, as a sacred and spiritual ceremony, the procedures are intended to be kept secret until such time as any individual student trains to be a Reiki Master. The second, less obvious reason is that when someone has their eyes closed, any external distractions around them are reduced, so that they are more easily able to stay in an appropriate meditative state, which leaves them more open to receive a mystical experience.

Experiencing an Attunement

Because Reiki is guided by a Higher Intelligence (the Source/God/All That Is) through your Higher Self, it adjusts to suit each person, so everyone's experience of a Reiki attunement is slightly different, even though the process carried out by the Reiki Master will be identical for everyone. If someone has already been doing energy work for some time—perhaps tai chi, chi gung or martial arts—or if they already do some form of spiritual healing, then their bodies are already tuned in to higher energetic vibrations, so they are able to "absorb" more Reiki right from the moment they are attuned. The same is often true of people who have done quite a lot of spiritual work, including deep meditation. However, if a person has never done anything in terms of energy or spiritual work, they will still be able to channel Reiki, but initially the flow of energy they experience may be less intense. After a few weeks of practice, however, there is very little difference between the amount of Reiki flowing through the energetically or spiritually experienced person, and someone who was previously inexperienced.

At each *level* of attunement (Reiki 1, 2 or 3) you become able to tap into a higher, wider channel of that universal energy, and the vibrationary rate of your energy body is increased. After an attunement is over, students often describe the beautiful spiritual or mystical experiences they have received, such as "seeing" wonderful colors, visions or past life experiences. Others report receiving personal messages or profound healing, sensing the presence of guides or angelic beings, or simply having a feeling of complete peace. Some people go through a real shift in their awareness immediately afterward, describing the sensation as almost like being reborn, so that they experience everything around them more intensely—colors are brighter, their sense of smell is enhanced, and sounds are sharper. Others feel a buzzing or heightened sensitivity in the crown center for a short while, or describe a sense of floating or light-headedness. All of these reactions are absolutely normal—but so is experiencing very little sensation, or even nothing at all, which may be a bit disappointing for some students. However, an attunement always works, 100 percent success rate, all of the time. This is what is so exciting—it is *not possible* to fail a Reiki course, provided a qualified Reiki Master carries out the attunement process with you. You *will* be able to channel Reiki. But you won't necessarily feel anything, at least at first.

AN ENERGETIC CHANNEL

Being initiated into Reiki is therefore a powerful spiritual experience, and it is the attunement process that provides one of the major differences between Reiki and other "hands-on healing" methods, such as traditional spiritual healing. The energetic channel that is reopened during the spiritual empowerment becomes active immediately, so within minutes you can begin to draw Reiki through yourself, and use it either for your own healing, or to heal other people, animals, and so on. From then on, whenever you intend to use Reiki, simply thinking about it, or holding your hands out in readiness to use it, will activate it—there are no complicated rituals to follow.

This "instant" acquisition of healing ability is one of the

things that makes Reiki so unique, but is probably also the most puzzling aspect of it to Western minds. We are not used to anything so valuable being achieved so effortlessly, yet, as mentioned, in the East spiritual empowerments are a well-known and accepted way of acquiring energy, knowledge, wisdom or insight. Interestingly, in an interview with the eminent scientist James L. Oschman, PhD, after explaining what a Reiki attunement was, one of my Reiki Masters, William Lee Rand, asked him whether there was any scientific explanation for such a transfer of ability. Oschman's answer was to hypothesize that " . . .what is being passed during the attunement process is a frequency or a set of frequencies that can be transferred from a teacher to a student via the energy field, and that will always be remembered by the student." He compared it to the memory process in homeopathy, in which an electromagnetic signature of a substance is transferred to water.

What the attunement process is creating is a permanent energetic channel in your energy body, through which Reiki (and only Reiki) can flow. The channel runs from your crown chakra, through your brow chakra and throat chakra to your heart chakra, and from there it runs down each arm to the chakra in the center of each palm.

This channel isn't visible (except perhaps to people with exceptional psychic gifts), but I always think of it as an energy equivalent of a fiber-optic tube. Just as light can flow down a fiber-optic tube, so Reiki can flow down the Reiki channel. Some Masters describe it as a pipe or conduit, which can be a useful analogy because with each attunement you receive the "conduit" becomes slightly bigger, and can channel more Reiki.

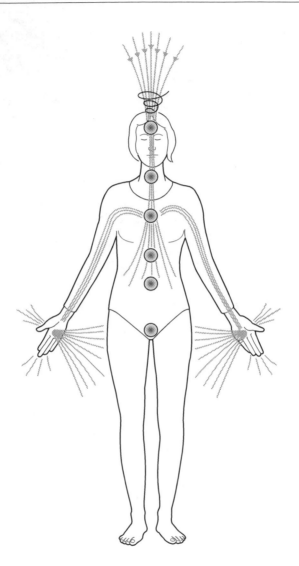

THE EFFECTS OF ATTUNEMENT TO REIKI

The attunement is only the *start* of your connection to Reiki, and over the ensuing weeks and months as you practice using it, the flow of Reiki gains strength, so that within six to eight weeks after being initiated into Reiki (at any level) you are experiencing the full flow of energy. Basically, the more you use it, the better it flows, and once you have received a Reiki attunement you will be able to use Reiki for the rest of your life—it won't wear off or wear out.

If for some reason you don't use Reiki for a number of years, you may *think* it isn't flowing because you don't have any sensation of it in your hands. Some people ask to be reattuned if this happens, but there really is no need, because it *is* still there. You just need to practice a bit to bring back the full flow. Of course, some students enjoy attunements so much that they want to repeat the experience as often as possible, which is one of the reasons why some people choose to progress very quickly through Reiki 1, 2 and 3. Other people choose instead to attend Reiki courses with several different Masters for the same level, sometimes because they are under the mistaken impression that they haven't been attuned "properly," or that because they haven't used their Reiki for months, or years, it won't work anymore. Some Reiki Masters are very much against this, but although I wouldn't wish to encourage people to become "attunement junkies," there is nothing intrinsically wrong with having a number of attunements at the same level, as each attunement helps to strengthen the Reiki channel, enabling even more Reiki to flow through. Indeed, in Japan it is usual for Reiki students to gather together about once a month with their Master to share experiences of doing self-treatments, giving treatments to others, asking questions, and receiving a simple form of attunement/empowerment called "Reiju," which increases the power and flow of the Reiki they can channel, and is beneficial for their spiritual development, too.

The more you use Reiki, and the further into Reiki you progress (i.e., taking further training and experiencing more attunements), the more the Reiki is able to clear your energy channels and pathways, and the easier it becomes for Reiki to raise your energetic vibrations to the next appropriate level. This effectively raises your consciousness, so that your connection with your Soul/Higher Self becomes closer, and therefore its guidance becomes more easily accessible to you. You may feel guided to meditate more, in order to explore aspects of spirituality that hadn't previously interested you. You may feel the need to let go of restrictions in your life that are stifling your personal and spiritual development, which might mean a need to change your job, see less of some friends, take more time for yourself despite family commitments, or end a relationship that has become unhealthy or oppressive.

Reiki can therefore lead you toward a deeper, more meaningful and fulfilling life. Reiki is an energy, a tool for healing, a vehicle for learning and a catalyst for change. It is a gift of incredible power and sometimes daunting complexity, but it is available to everyone, when they are ready.

chapter nine

DEVELOPMENTS IN WESTERN REIKI TRAINING

Until the early 1990s I suspect that most people attending Reiki courses experienced very similar theories and practices, but since then there have been many changes in the way Reiki is taught. Some of these modifications have been referred to in Chapter 7, such as the reduction in time between the three levels, and the change from apprenticeship to short courses for Master training, but there have been many other amendments over the past 20 years or so. For example, the fee structure that Mrs. Takata started is now only kept to by Masters who are members of the Reiki Alliance, so most people pay less to learn Reiki, especially at Master level, and the system is no longer regarded as a purely oral tradition, as most Masters now give out manuals or handouts to their students. We aren't sure why Takata taught the system as an oral tradition, as we now know that both Usui and Hayashi used instruction manuals in their classes.

THE USUI/TIBETAN REIKI SYSTEM

There are still only four symbols in the Usui system, but many Masters now teach the Usui/Tibetan system developed by William Lee Rand, which includes another two symbols. This is based on the traditional Usui Reiki, as taught by Mrs. Takata, but with additions such as scanning, beaming, meditation, psychic surgery (which he now calls aura clearing), healing attunements and acknowledgment of the role played by spiritual beings in the healing process. The attunement process is also different, incorporating a Tibetan technique that William developed after receiving inner guidance, and the system is taught in four levels rather than three—Reiki 1, Reiki 2, Advanced Reiki Training (ART) and Reiki Master.

Unfortunately, many Masters who use and attune people to this system of Reiki do not realize that it is not the traditional Usui Reiki, so the differences are becoming more and more blurred. Similarly, there are other lineages, such as Diane Stein's, which use additional symbols, but which are still described as Usui Reiki. It does sound like a bit of a minefield, I'll admit, but there is really no need to be concerned, as all the Reiki systems work, and whichever style you become attuned to, you will be able to channel some form of Reiki energy.

OTHER FORMS OF REIKI

So far I have mentioned Usui Reiki and Usui/Tibetan Reiki, but over the past 20 years many other healing systems have evolved, most of which use the word "Reiki" in their names. The most popular are probably Karuna Reiki, an additional system developed by American Reiki Master William Lee Rand using 12 symbols, which is only taught to people who are already qualified as Reiki Masters; and Tera Mai Seichem, a system developed by Kathleen Milner in the U.S.A. which utilizes some of the same symbols as Karuna Reiki, plus some others, and can be taught to people who have not learned any other system of Reiki. Both systems are available in the UK, U.S.A., Canada, Australia, New Zealand and many other countries.

There are, however, many more systems, some of which are easy to find, and some that now seem to be extinct. Others are only available in particular countries, such as India, but you can find out more about most of them on the Internet. Other Reiki systems include Ascension Reiki; Amanohuna Reiki; Blue Star Reiki; Brahma Satya Reiki; Buddho-Ennersense; Gendai Reiki Ho; Golden Age Reiki; Ichi Sekai Reiki; Jinlap Maitri Reiki; Johrei; Mari-el; Medicine Dharma Reiki; New Life Reiki; The Radiance Technique (also known as Authentic Reiki and Real Reiki); Raku Kei Reiki; Reiki-ho; Reiki Jin-Kei Do; Reiki Plus; Saku Reiki; Satya Japanese Reiki; Sekhem; Shambhala Reiki; Sun Li Chung Reiki; Usuido Reiki and Vajra Reiki.

This may not be an exhaustive list, as new names seem to crop up quite often, but most of them are based at least loosely on the original Usui Reiki, so if you are interested it may be worth you doing some research to see if any of them appeal to you.

TECHNIQUES FROM JAPAN

Another major change since the late 1990s has been the inclusion of some of Usui's original techniques from Japan either as part of a Reiki 1 or Reiki 2 course, or presented as a separate workshop. At present only a fairly small proportion of Reiki Masters seems to know these methods, but this knowledge is spreading, so do ask any potential Masters you might wish to train with whether they include any of the following in their training:

- Original Usui hand positions on the head (see Chapter 10).
- Hatsurei-ho—a combined meditation and cleansing technique (see Chapter 11) including Gassho, a meditation posture.
- Byosen Reikan-ho—scanning by feeling resonance or sensations in the hand to detect places which need Reiki.
- Reiji-ho—an advanced scanning technique, allowing Reiki to guide you to a place that needs healing.
- Nen-tatsu-ho—a technique to cleanse negative thoughts and emotions.
- Jaki Kiri Joka-ho—a technique to purify negative energy in objects.
- Tanden Chiryo-ho—a detoxifying technique.
- Heso Chiryo-ho—a deep-healing technique based at the navel.
- Uchite Chiryo-ho—patting gently with the hands.
- Oshite Chiryo-ho—pushing gently with the fingers.
- Nadete Chiryo-ho—stroking gently with the hands.
- Koki-ho—using the breath for healing.

◆ Gyoshi-ho—using the eyes for healing.
◆ Reiki Mawashi—sharing Reiki in a group circle.
◆ Shuchu Reiki—a group treatment.
◆ Renzoku Reiki—a Reiki marathon (taking it in turns to treat someone constantly over a period of time).

There are instructions for using many of the above techniques in my book *Reiki For Life*, if you would like to know more.

AREAS OF CONCERN

In the twenty-first century other ways of acquiring the ability to channel Reiki are now being explored, such as receiving an attunement at a distance and/or over the Internet, with either correspondence courses as a backup, or no formal instruction at all. Very recently one or two books have been published that give instruction on how to attune yourself without attending a class or even logging on to the Internet.

Distant Attunements

I try really hard not to be judgmental about anything that is done in the name of Reiki, but the issue of distant attunements, and carrying out self-attunements from instructions in a book, is a thorny one. There is no doubt that distant attunements will work, because there are no barriers to energy—we don't think it strange that our TVs and radios work, despite the fact that the source of the signals is a long way away. I decided I couldn't really judge them until I'd experienced one, so I chose a respected Reiki Master in Canada to carry one out on me, and I certainly felt it, although not as strongly as an in-person attunement.

As I see it, the main problems with distant attunements are, a) that the student doesn't have the same opportunities as they would in a class, to receive knowledge and instruction, ask questions, practice treatments, understand what Reiki is and does, etc., and b) it could potentially downgrade the credibility of Reiki. It is difficult enough now to convince skeptics, especially in the medical field, that Reiki is beneficial, because they don't believe that anything good can be learned so quickly and easily. But that's when they know it can be achieved in a few days. If they find out you can get it "over the Internet" in moments, bang goes our reputation! However, perhaps that's just our human perception, linked to our human fears. I doubt if Reiki is bothered "how" people tune in to the energy, and I am sure that the Reiki Masters who carry out distant attunements believe that what they are doing is right. Their motivations seem generally to be to spread Reiki as far as possible, and are rarely to do with money, as they often offer attunements for free, or for a very low price. However, many of them seem to recommend that someone who has done no Reiki previously should be attuned straightaway at Master level, and I do take issue with that. To understand why, read Chapter 16—there are good reasons for progressing through the levels.

Self-attunements

Metaphysically it is probably quite possible to carry out a self-attunement, although this isn't something I can personally check out, because someone else has already attuned me. However, some people naturally develop the ability to channel healing energy, sometimes as young children, sometimes as adults, without going through any training course or attunement process. Indeed, this may even be a development in Reiki linked to the raising in consciousness of so many people who have already been attuned in the traditional way—the global energetic vibrations now are very different from those of 10, 20, 30 or more years ago.

The "teacher" in me isn't very happy with either of these developments, I'll admit, because I don't think they are the "best" way of acquiring Reiki. I am something of a traditionalist, and Suzuki-san, one of Dr. Usui's original students (see page 20), was quite firm in stating that Reiki should only be passed on "in person," so I go along with that. Also, I suppose that as an educationalist, I like to uphold and encourage high standards of teaching, which in turn can (but don't always) result in high standards of learning. We have seen so many changes in the past 20 years in the way Reiki is taught, and each time something "new" turns up it rattles our cages, disturbs our comfort zones—so perhaps the main point is that all the changes we've seen have actually resulted in more and more people being able to do Reiki. From my perspective that's a good thing, even if I wouldn't personally use some of the methods. We're all allowed to be a bit different!

TRAINING AS A REIKI PRACTITIONER IN THE UK

Perhaps one of the biggest changes, at least in the UK, is fairly recent. When I originally wrote this book in 2006, a consultation document was being made available through the various Reiki organizations (see Resources) to everyone who does Reiki, regarding voluntary self-regulation (VSR).

In 2003, a number of Reiki organizations in the UK met to discuss the possibility of voluntary self-regulation, rather than potentially having regulation imposed upon us by government in the future. They agreed to work together so that progress could be made on identifying consistent, high professional standards, and in the development of a single UK register for professional Reiki practitioners, and a single regulatory body. This initial meeting led to the establishment of the Reiki Regulatory Working Group (RRWG) with the remit to develop a definition of minimum standards that could be applied to all Reiki groups, allowing for variation in styles, to prepare a safe code of professional practice of Reiki, including disciplinary and complaints procedures, and to set up a national register of Reiki practitioners and teachers. This work has been supported by the influential Princes' Foundation for Integrated Health (PFIH).

I was pleased to be a member of the RRWG education and accreditation subcommittee that drafted the majority of these proposals, so I know that the RRWG was totally committed to the preservation of Reiki as a spiritual practice and healing art, and they respect and honor all styles and traditions of Reiki. The regulatory process is about looking after clients' needs, not about regulating the practitioners' individual style of practice. However, now in 2012 there is the opportunity for those wishing to practice Reiki professionally to work through an education and accreditation process in order to become UK-registered Reiki practitioners on a national register. I will discuss this more fully in Chapter 15, because in essence it will affect only those people who want to practice professionally, although the register will provide an excellent resource for people wanting to find a qualified practitioner.

In order to encompass all "styles" of Reiki, it was suggested that education requirements will not be set at any particular "level" or "degree," but on the following:

♦ Having been connected to Reiki in person by a Reiki teacher (a minimum of one in-person attunement/ initiation is already in the Reiki National Occupational Standards).
♦ A minimum number of hours learning and practice.
♦ The ability to comply with the Reiki National Occupational Standards.
♦ A commitment to personal practice.

There will therefore have to be some fairly major changes in the future in the way in which professional Reiki practitioners will be trained, but I would emphasize again that no changes will be required for people who just want to use Reiki on themselves, or their friends or family. They can continue to take Reiki courses with whichever Reiki Master they feel drawn to, as they have always done. For some general guidance about what will be required of a professional practitioner, see Chapter 15.

THE NEXT STEP—USING REIKI

In Part 4, we look at some of the ways in which you can use Reiki for your own healing and protection, as well as for personal and spiritual growth, and at how it can be used creatively, including in working with animals, which I know is a popular topic with many people interested in Reiki.

part four

USING REIKI

chapter ten

SELF-HEALING AND
SELF-TREATING

Self-healing is a lifelong process of taking responsibility
for your own health and well-being by treating yourself—and particularly your body—with love and respect.
It also means making the most of your personal potential
by taking a holistic view of yourself and trying to live in
the best way possible for you. This means developing an
awareness of your whole self, so to take a holistic view,
self-healing is to do with health in any area of our lives—
physical, emotional, mental, spiritual and even environmental.

SELF-HEALING WITH REIKI

Self-healing is one of the most important aspects of
Reiki at all levels, and is certainly the major focus of
Reiki at First Degree. It is an act of self-love to give
yourself a Reiki treatment every day, to give yourself that
priority, to find the time to just "be" with yourself, and
because Reiki works holistically, it will also support any

other aspects of your self-healing program. However, doing a self-treatment is only part of the story. Reiki works holistically, and your use of it helps healing to take place in each of the four bodies—physical, emotional, mental and spiritual—for the rest of your life. After you have been using Reiki for some months you will proba-bly start to be aware that other healing effects are begin-ning to happen.

Physical

You are likely to become much more aware of your physical body and what it needs, and it is important to listen to your body's messages and to actively follow up on what you have learned, making the necessary changes to the way you think and act in relation to your physical health. How do you use your physical body in terms of exercise, awareness and touch? What is the importance to you of food and drink, sex, being outdoors, being in the countryside and being connected with the elements (air, water, fire and earth)?

What is your body image? Do you like your body? You need to work on clearing out any negative self-beliefs, such as thinking you are too fat, too thin, too tall or too short. Start accepting and loving your body, appreciating it for the fine job it does, praising it instead of complain-ing about it, and giving it the priority in your life that it deserves.

A number of therapies have stimulating yet relaxing effects on the body, and could become part of your self-healing program alongside Reiki. These include aro-matherapy, massage, reflexology and shiatsu, and gentle exercises such as tai chi and yoga.

Emotional

You will begin to discover more about your emotional body, which reacts to every emotion you experience, so it makes sense to work on releasing negative feelings such as anger, jealousy, resentment or guilt, and replacing them with positive ones such as love, compassion, freedom and happiness (you could use the visualization on page 117 to help with this). Try to spend as little time as possible in negative situations or with negative people, and work at improving all your relationships, from partner and family, to friends and colleagues.

How do you use your emotional energy? What fears are you working through—fear of death, fear of being left out, fear of rejection, fear of loss, fear of change, etc.? How can you open to more joy in your life and learn to express your emotions more easily? Of course it is important to acknowledge your feelings, so learning to express them sensitively but effectively will help to harness the more creative, positive energy of your emotions.

What can you do to improve the important relationships in your life? How can you achieve a better relationship with yourself? Work on loving yourself totally and absolutely—but start simply by accepting yourself, just as you are, and the liking and the loving will come more naturally. Do things you enjoy, build some creativity into your life, give yourself treats, and simply have some fun.

There may be other practical steps you can take to improve your emotional health. Sometimes we need outside help to sort things out, so experiencing some counseling, psychotherapy or hypnotherapy might be a good step forward. Other methods you could explore are neuro-linguistic programming (NLP), transactional

153

analysis (TA), family therapy, or some of the newer procedures such as emotional freedom technique (EFT) or
Tapas acupressure technique (TAT)—see page 157 for
definitions, and page 281 for useful resources. You can
also use visualizations and affirmations, in addition to
Reiki, to help with emotional problems.

Mental

Another effect of using Reiki is likely to be acquiring
more understanding of your mental body. Your thought
energy is what creates your life, attracting to you the
things you think about, so it is vital to use your mind
constructively and positively, acknowledging and then
letting go of negative thoughts. The key is to live in the
present, rather than in the past or future. It would be useful to spend some time reviewing your thought patterns,
beliefs, attitudes and concepts, and to let go of those that
are no longer useful to you, such as prejudice, intoler-
ance, bigotry or judgmental criteria. Do your best to cut
down on the stress in your life, whether it is home or
work based, by developing a more laid-back approach.
Most of us get bogged down in trivia for 80 percent of
our time, spending only 20 percent on what is really
important. So prioritize everything you have to do and
practice good time management. You'll release lots of
time for things you want to do, so you can develop the
habit of giving time to yourself for enjoyable pursuits, or
just "quiet time."

Ask yourself whether you are able to use your mind to
further your goals, or whether your mind is constantly in
the way of you getting things done. Are you experiencing too much guilt about the past, too much worry

about the future? Are you going over and over things in your mind? Look at how you can bring more relaxation and peaceful contemplation into your life.

Practical steps to relaxation, which is the key to a stable and rested mental body, are plenty of sleep and regular meditation (only about 15 minutes a day are needed, see page 175). Also, treating yourself occasionally to some of the therapies I've already mentioned, such as an aromatherapy massage or a reflexology treatment, will be helpful, and you might also find Bach Flower Remedies, visualizations and NLP useful.

Spiritual

The development of spiritual awareness gives your life meaning, so perhaps you need to examine your attitudes to spirituality and religion. What are your personal ideas about life and death? What are your feelings about other people's beliefs? Do you feel happy to develop your own personal spiritual beliefs, or would you feel more comfortable exploring different religions until you found something that felt right?

How important is your spiritual life? Are you focused on it, or does your "everyday life" intrude so much that your spirituality is continually on the "back burner"? Begin to look at your soul's journey into the light and at the path of your spiritual evolution. How might you evolve more, spiritually? What can you do to "connect" more, to pursue your own path to enlightenment? You might want to spend more time in meditation, or simply in quiet contemplation, or reading spiritually uplifting books. Sound healing (e.g., chanting, toning, drumming, Tibetan bowls), creative pursuits such as painting or writing, and spending time with nature can also help to bring you into a more peaceful, loving and spiritual "space."

Environmental

Gradually, as you integrate your physical, emotional, mental and spiritual bodies, you will begin to realize that your whole being is impacted by the world around you. You will want to be surrounded more by beauty and clear energies, and may want to spend more time outdoors, especially in the countryside, where the air and energy are fresher and clearer—but you will want your home to reflect these values, too, so you might like to explore the theories of feng shui (for books, see page 287).

You might become more interested in environmental issues such as recycling waste, growing food organically, saving woods and forests for future generations, keeping rivers and seas unpolluted, and so on. You may also develop concerns about the growing electromagnetic pollution from cell phones, TV, radio and satellite signals, overhead electricity cables and the many pieces of electrical equipment most of us have in our homes. The World Health Organization (WHO) cites that humans today are potentially being bombarded with up to 20,000 times more electromagnetic pollution than our prehistoric ancestors!

This is a form of geopathic stress, and the word "geopathic" comes from the Greek "geo," meaning "of the earth," and "pathos," which describes suffering or disease. There are a variety of sources for geopathic energy, such as the earth's magnetic field, which includes earth energies such as ley lines. In addition, natural disturbances like geological faults, ore masses and underground water can affect us, too, although it is human-made disturbances that tend to have the greatest effect. These include mining and underground utilities, as well as the overhead power lines and electronic signals already mentioned.

There's not much we can do about naturally occurring energies, but if possible, avoid living in places near to overhead cables or power-generating equipment, don't have electrical equipment, such as TVs or radio-alarm clocks, in your bedroom, and switch off all electrical appliances at the socket unless you are using them.

In every case, you can use Reiki to help—you can even regularly write down on paper any problem area you are working on, hold the paper between your hands and send it Reiki.

DEFINITIONS

Neuro-Linguistic Programming (NLP)

NLP was begun in the midseventies by a linguist, John Grinder, and a mathematician, Richard Bandler, who had strong interests in successful people, psychology, language and computer programming. They developed a range of communication and persuasion techniques, including self-hypnosis, to help people to motivate and change themselves, and create greater self-esteem, by reprogramming their brains. At another level, NLP is about self-discovery, exploring identity and mission. It also provides a framework for understanding and relating to the "spiritual" part of human experience that reaches beyond us as individuals to our family, community and global systems.

Transactional Analysis (TA)

Eric Berne, the founder of TA, developed the theory of TA, based on theories of personality and social psychology within the humanistic tradition. He identified three "ego states," the parent, adult and child, which he believed coexist in all people. TA offers a framework for understanding personality, human development, communications and personal life patterns, and it provides ways to describe and explain both internal experience and interpersonal behavior in an innovative and accessible manner.

Emotional Freedom Technique (EFT)

This is a form of "emotional acupressure." Dr. Roger Callahan, a clinical psychologist, is credited with discovering that tapping with a finger on specific acupuncture/acupressure points, while focusing one's attention on a problem, removes the emotional component. EFT works by removing the negative emotional factor from a memory, event, circumstance or situation. Negative emotions can be a disruption in the body's energy circuits, so learning and using this technique removes distress within your body, and this can have a profound and pleasing effect on attitudes, perception, relationships and even health.

Tapas Acupressure Technique (TAT)

Similar to EFT (see above), TAT is a simple technique based on applying gentle pressure on certain acupuncture points on the face and back of the head to attain a feeling of relaxation and empowerment. It can also be used to help against phobias, allergies and emotional issues.

BALANCING YOUR LIFE AND YOUR BODY WITH REIKI

Bringing Reiki into yourself regularly begins the process of dislodging blocks and obstacles within your energetic system, and as they are dislodged and removed they come to the surface for review. This often means that memories of past events suddenly come into your mind, or you start to have very vivid dreams. You don't need to become overly identified with them when this happens; simply acknowledge them and let them go. (Imagining them in a pink bubble, and seeing that bubble rise up into the sky and beyond, to the universe, is a good way to release them.) Occasionally you may even find that old situations recur, so you might feel that all those old problems have come back to plague you! At this stage the temptation is to discontinue your self-treatments, because you are afraid they are making things worse. However, you need to understand that this is a necessary part of the process, and that you can use Reiki to heal, harmonize and balance these old feelings and fears simply by *intending* that this should happen. Presently you will feel better than you have ever felt before, as you rid yourself of years of blocked or stagnant energy.

If there are a great many blockages to clear, you may very occasionally experience physical reactions when you are treating yourself, such as trembling and shaking. Usually this dissipates quickly, but if it becomes too uncomfortable, discontinue the treatment for a few minutes and breathe deeply. If the trembling doesn't immediately stop, you could try grounding yourself by stamping vigorously on the floor for about 20 to 30 seconds, or do the Cross Crawl exercise (see page 84).

REIKI HAND POSITIONS FOR SELF-TREATMENT

The Reiki hand positions for a self-treatment are basically the same as those for treating other people (see page 71), and once you have practiced them for a while you will find it easy to remember their order. Each hand position should feel comfortable, and should usually be held for between two and five minutes, depending upon how much time you are able to allocate to a self-treatment. In terms of timing, I find it easiest to count the seconds silently—it turns the treatment into a type of meditation, and in any case, I prefer to keep my eyes closed, so I can't see a clock. If any area appears to need longer (i.e., your hands are still reacting with heat or tingling), then it is fine to continue for as long as seems appropriate.

There are various ways of keeping to set times for each hand position; I recently began to use a lovely pyramid-shaped meditation timer which sounds a soft gong every 2½, 3, 4, 5 or 10 minutes—I can set it for as long as I wish—details are on my website. Alternatively there are CDs of music designed for Reiki treatments that also sound a gong every five minutes, or simply have a gap in the music. You could even make your own CDs or tapes, using your choice of gentle music. However, the timing is less important than just giving yourself Reiki, so even if you have very little time, one minute in each hand position is better than not doing it at all.

All the same, you should consider why you cannot give yourself enough time to do a self-treatment. If you gave each hand position about two and a half minutes the whole treatment would take only half an hour. Are you living life at too hectic a pace? Are you giving your needs too little priority, rushing around after everyone else instead? Giving Reiki to yourself is giving yourself love—and you deserve love, don't you? (If you mentally replied "no" to that question, then you really need to work with Reiki on your issues of self-love!)

A FULL SELF-TREATMENT

A full self-treatment can be carried out with you lying down or sitting in a chair, and it starts with four or five hand positions on the head, then four on the front of the body, finishing with four on the back of the body. It is optional to give Reiki to the thighs, knees, calves, ankles and feet, or to the upper arms, elbows, forearms, wrists, hands or fingers, but if you have a health problem there, it makes sense to treat it. Also, you may like to begin with some self-scanning, to identify any areas on your body that may be in particular need of Reiki.

Self-scanning

Gently draw your hand down the front of your body, from the crown of your head to your pelvic area—or further, down to your feet—sensing any variations in the feel of the energy on your hand, and make a mental note of which places seem to need more Reiki.

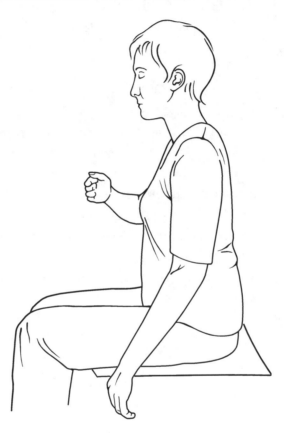

Positions on the Head

You can start with either both of your hands on the crown of your head, or place one hand on the crown and one at the back of the head, as shown here.

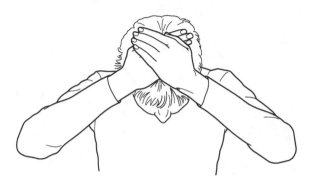

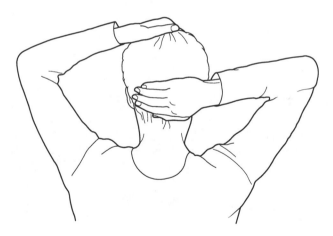

The order of the next three positions isn't vital—some people like to treat the eyes, then the ears, then the back of the head—but just do them in whatever order feels right and comfortable for you.

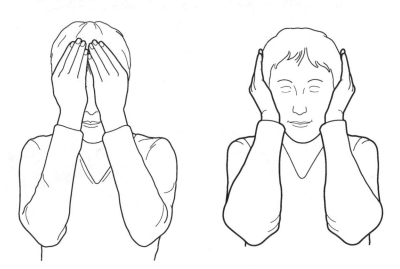

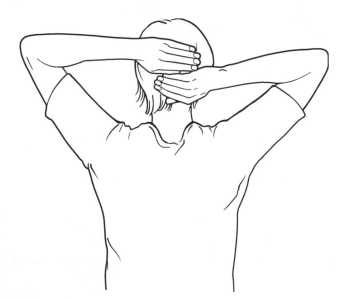

When you move your hands down to the throat, there are several ways in which you can position them.

Hand Positions for the Front of the Body

There are normally four positions on the front of the body—the chest, solar plexus, navel area and pelvic area. On the chest there are a couple of ways you can place your hands, as shown in the illustrations.

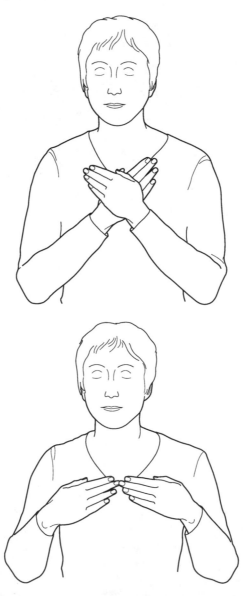

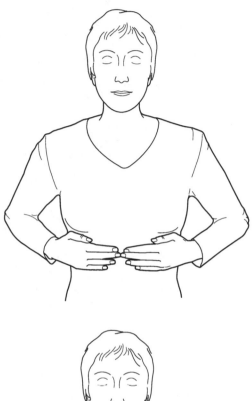

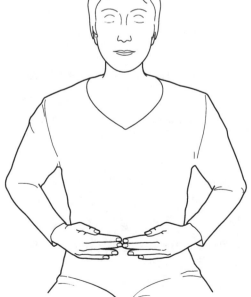

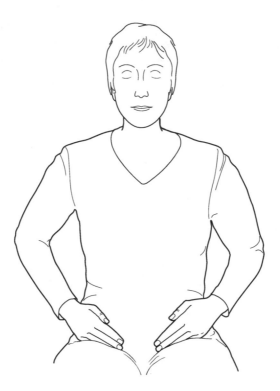

Hand Positions for the Back of the Body

The four hand positions on the back of the body start with the shoulders, and there are several ways you can do this, depending upon which you find most comfortable. The positions down the rest of the back can be a little more difficult, unless you are quite flexible, so feel free to place the backs of your hands against your body, rather than the palms, if that feels easier and more comfortable— the palm chakra allows Reiki to flow out of both sides of the hand, so you'll get the same benefits either way.

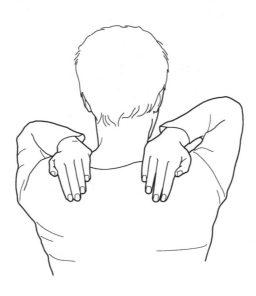

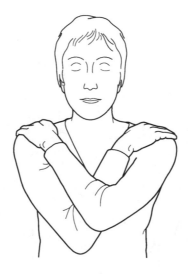

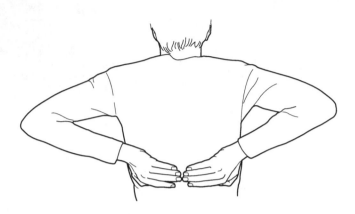

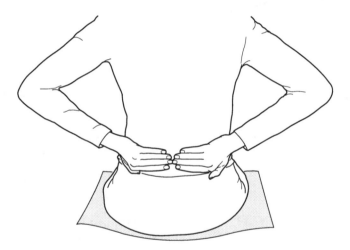

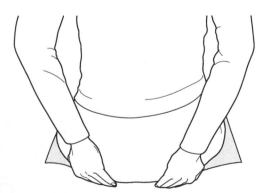

OTHER WAYS OF SELF-TREATING

You may not always have the time or be in the right place to carry out a full self-treatment, so you might like to carry out the shorter self-treatment, which was apparently used by Dr. Usui. It concentrates on the head, and you can hold each hand position for between three and five minutes—or longer, if you wish.

Zento-bu Place your hand on top of your forehead, between your eyebrows and the line where your hair starts to grow.

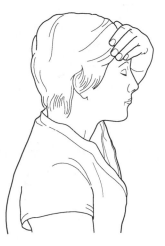

Koutou-bu Place your hand at the back of your head, roughly at the middle point between the top of your head and the top of your spine.

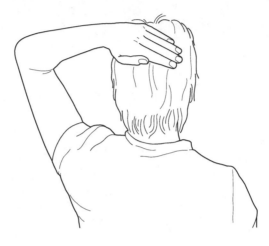

Enzui-bu Place your hand at the base of the skull, where the brain and spine meet.

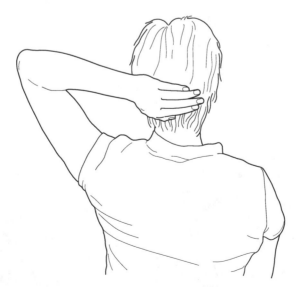

Sokuto-bu Place one hand on each of your temples.

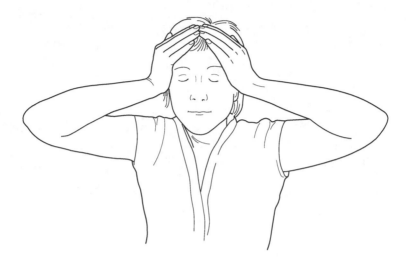

Touchu-bu Place your hand right at the top of your head, on your crown.

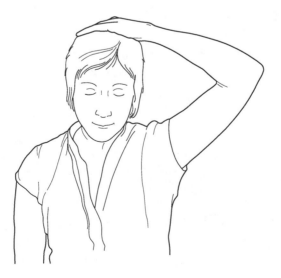

REIKI AS FIRST AID

Of course, when you need some Reiki you don't always have to carry out a full self-treatment, or even the shorter Usui self-treatment. Perhaps you have a headache—just place your hands anywhere on your head for as long as it takes for the pain to go away. Maybe you've banged your elbow on a cupboard—cradle it with your other hand and let the Reiki flow. Or you've suddenly got a cramp in your leg—place both hands on the affected area until shortly after the muscles become relaxed again. Whenever you have a pain or injury you can give it Reiki for as long as you want, and it will help to accelerate the healing process and reduce the pain.

TAKING RESPONSIBILITY FOR YOUR HEALTH AND WELL-BEING

I believe we need to develop an "attitude of gratitude" for our physical bodies as the vehicles we have chosen to live in for this life. Like any vehicle, your body needs good maintenance, some tender loving care and a few words of appreciation now and then to keep it running sweetly! Giving yourself Reiki every day will certainly help, but it doesn't make you invincible. You can still be vulnerable to ill health if you don't look after yourself. Eating in an unhealthy way, drinking too much alcohol, smoking or taking "recreational" drugs, never exercising, not getting enough sleep and leading a very stressful life—any or all of these things are likely to lead to poor health.

Taking responsibility for your own health means acting

responsibly, so take a look at the way you live and see if you can institute some improvements. Eating a balanced diet of mainly fresh foods (i.e., not processed), including at least five portions of vegetables and fruit each day, drinking plenty of water, taking some exercise such as walking, cycling or swimming at least three times a week, and getting seven or eight hours sleep most nights of the week, will make you feel—and probably look—better. If you also limit your consumption of alcohol, and preferably give up smoking and nonprescription drugs, that will help a lot, too, and if you can de-stress your life, perhaps by including some meditation, breathing and relaxation techniques, or creative pursuits in your life, that will build in levels of fulfillment which will increase your chances of good health.

Reiki is wonderful, and it can do the most miraculous and amazing things, but it still needs a willingness on the part of the person receiving the Reiki—a readiness to allow changes in lifestyle, in attitude, in ways of being—so that the healing can be completed and fully integrated into that person's life. So being good to yourself by giving yourself Reiki every day, and by adopting a healthier lifestyle, can give you the optimum chance of achieving or maintaining a healthy body.

THE BENEFITS OF MEDITATION

Meditation has been medically proved to be really beneficial, as it helps to lower both your heart rate and blood pressure. In all forms of meditation there is a focus and a quieting of the mind. This aims at first simply to reduce, and eventually to eliminate, the chatter of daily life, and the stresses of the environment in which we live, and so provide a haven within which we are free to connect with our inner being. It helps us to overcome the problems and illusions we create for ourselves and that we allow others to create for us, and also to overcome habits we have formed that hold us back. Meditation allows us to go beyond the everyday, into who we really are. The art of focusing, and awareness of being in the moment, changes brain activity, which leads to deep relaxation and a sense of joy.

One of the problems with meditation is that people think it is difficult, but actually it can be as simple as just being quiet and letting your thoughts drift, perhaps while sitting in the garden, or by a lake or river, or even in your living room. The confusion probably comes from a misunderstanding, the idea that you have to completely empty your mind when meditating. Well, yes, that is the eventual aim, but it could take 10, 20 or even 30 years of practice before you get to that stage, so don't be put off. You might consider signing up for meditation classes, which are often available at your local college or Buddhist center.

chapter eleven

ENERGETIC CLEANSING AND PROTECTION

Knowledge about energetic protection and cleansing was not included in any Reiki training in the West, as far as we know, until the late 1990s. It is possible that Mrs. Takata did mention it to her students but because she taught Reiki as an oral system, and possibly because as Westerners they didn't understand energy in the way they do in the East, it was simply forgotten, or was not deemed to be very important. However, since more information has come out of Japan about Usui and his original system it is clear that, as a martial arts expert, he would have been well acquainted with energy, so some of the cleansing techniques that were used in his original system are based on the Japanese version of chi kung, known as Ki-kou. There are good reasons for using some form of energetic cleansing and protection on a daily basis, and including them in your everyday healing routines will have a positive effect on your energy levels, health and well-being.

WHY DO WE NEED ENERGY CLEANSING AND PROTECTION?

As I have explained in Chapter 4, everything is energy, and energies can have negative, positive or sometimes neutral vibrations. Being attuned to Reiki raises your body's vibrations, and as the energetic oscillations become faster, this makes your whole energy field lighter and less dense as you gradually become more and more "enlightened." This not only increases your spiritual awareness, but also means that your whole energy field can become more permeable, and therefore potentially more vulnerable to denser energies, which are attracted to the light.

This happens because as your energies become lighter and vibrate faster, there is more "space" between the energy particles, which the denser, negative energies could attempt to fill. As an analogy, imagine placing pebbles in a bowl until it is full—it appears to be completely filled, but if you poured water into the bowl, the water would occupy the space between the pebbles. It is therefore essential to cleanse and protect your entire energy field regularly, because otherwise it could become clogged with negative energy from outside sources, and if it becomes too blocked there is the possibility that this could manifest as illness.

SOURCES OF NEGATIVE ENERGY

The sources are many and varied, and can be physical energy, mental or thought energy, emotional energy or spiritual energy. Newspapers, TV, radio and films often have sad, disturbing or horrific images and words, which can impact negatively on our energy fields, because we react to them mentally and emotionally, so it is important to be discriminating about what you read, watch and listen to. It is far better to be uplifted by beautiful music or happy, fun programs than to be dragged down by horror films or the negative stuff that is usually presented as "news."

Energy disturbances or blockages in other people's energy fields can impact us, including negative thoughts and emotions, and negative blockages such as physical or mental illness, so our energies can be lowered when we spend time with negative people—you've probably encountered some people who seem to "drain" you when you are with them. Places can also impact our energies, especially if we spend time where negative energy can collect, such as shopping centers, city streets, offices and other workplaces, doctors' offices, hospitals, and even potentially our own home or homes belonging to friends and family. It would be a rare home indeed in which no conflict or argument or sorrow had ever happened, and disturbing mental and emotional energy can hang around for quite a long time.

Essentially, your beautiful, sparkling, clear and "enlightened" energy body can act like a sponge, mopping up the negative energy soup around you on a daily basis. Not exactly a happy thought, is it? But there's no need to panic—most of us do manage to cope pretty well with reasonable levels of negative energy, at least for quite some time, but it is sensible to be aware of them, and to carry out some protective activities, and some energy-cleansing activities, to ensure our maximum well-being.

Psychic Interference

Other things that could potentially affect your energy field negatively are psychic attack or being close to someone who is a psychic drain, and in rare cases there is also the possibility that you may encounter a field of evil energy, or that energetic entities might attach themselves to you. However, you can be reassured that most people don't encounter this sort of thing, but it is best to be prepared and know how to deal with it than to be unprepared and driven to panic. The first line of defense is not to be fearful—"light" always overcomes "dark."

Psychic Attack

This is basically harmful thoughts directed at you from other people, whether they are doing this consciously or not, and which can sometimes come in dreams—and thought energy can be a very powerful weapon in the wrong hands.

Psychic Drains

These are people whose own energy is low and so they drain your energy by "sucking" it into their own energy field, although many psychic drains are not actually aware that they are doing this. You might come across someone doing this on purpose, but this is pretty rare.

Evil Energy Fields

These exist because of a certain kind of human behavior, often held in places where torturous destruction of life has been done with a sense of pleasure, such as at the concentration camps in Nazi Germany, or the "killing fields" in Vietnam, although smaller areas of evil energy can be held in houses where awful things have happened, or in "seedy" nightclubs or similar places.

Entities

These are a bit more difficult to describe. They are supposed to be lower types of energy that have collected into a form (like a blob of consciousness, but the size can vary), which have absorbed some of the energy released by evil and negative human behavior, and can attach to a human energy field and "feed" off it so that it can continue its existence. They are attracted to negativity, but also to the shadow side of people intent on spiritual growth—religious history is full of people who dedicated themselves to the divine yet found themselves tormented by devils and demons. Occasionally they can be "ghosts"—i.e., the spirit form of a human who has lived on the earth plane, but hasn't yet gone "to the light," partly because they haven't yet acknowledged that they are "dead."

ENERGETIC PROTECTION

The first thing to do is to develop the habit of protecting yourself energetically every day, which doesn't have to be complicated. You can use your thought energy (which is very powerful) to visualize protective barriers around you, and of course you can use Reiki, with or without the symbols. A sensible way to use these methods is to carry out one or more of them every morning, especially before leaving home, although you can also use them at any time you feel particularly threatened, for example when going into some stressful situation or if you have to deal with very negative people in either a work or social situation.

- At Reiki 1, you can imagine yourself in a bubble of white or golden light that is above, below and on all sides of you, and is filled with Reiki; the edges of the bubble are permeable only by love, light, Reiki and positive energies. (If you haven't done a Reiki course yet, just imagine the bubble filled with white or golden light, and *intend* that it protects you.)
- If you have done Reiki 2, draw a large power symbol in front of you and step into it, saying its mantra three times. Imagine being wrapped inside the power symbol so that it is in front, behind and on each side of you, and *intend* that the Reiki protect you from any negativity or harm.
- Imagine yourself inside a bubble of Reiki light, and imagine that the bubble is closely surrounded by a fine mesh made of gold that is only permeable by love, light, Reiki and positive energies.
- If you ever feel really threatened, then do all of the above. Outside your bubble of light filled with Reiki and covered with gold mesh, imagine a ring of fire, and outside that imagine a shiny eggshell made of mirror or shiny silver, with the mirrored side facing outward. This effectively forms an energetic boundary around you, so that any negativity or psychic attack sent your way will only rebound

back to the sender, because it is reflected by the mirrored surface.

♦ Another method of self-protection if you feel really threatened is to fill your bubble with protective images such as a cross, a Star of David, the Hindu symbol for Om, or images of Jesus, Buddha or Kuan Yin.

♦ Imagine a circular shield over your solar plexus—it can be any size you need from a few inches up to 6 feet in diameter or more, which would then protect the whole of you. You can imagine the shield decorated with your favorite protective symbol, such as a cross.

♦ Imagine yourself as a flame, burning vibrantly, so that bad thoughts or feelings simply burn up when they come near you.

♦ Imagine yourself covered by a wonderful magic cloak and draw it around you. You can imagine it in any color, but perhaps you'd also like to imagine it with lots of Reiki symbols on it in gold or silver.

♦ Imagine each of your chakras as a flower, and simply close all the petals until they are tightly shut.

♦ Imagine a curtain hanging between you and the other person, from floor to ceiling, and gradually strengthen the curtain until you sense that it is made of lead, so that the other person's vibrations simply will not penetrate.

♦ Ask for help from your spirit guides and angels, if you are happy to accept that they exist.

Each of the above methods is useful in different situations, so use your intuition to decide which is the most appropriate at any particular time.

ENERGETIC CLEANSING

Dr. Usui is believed to have used a number of energetic cleansing methods as part of his healing system, and it is not necessary to use the Reiki symbols when carrying out any of them, so anyone with any level of Reiki can use them. However, if you have Second Degree you can enhance the process by drawing a power symbol over each hand before you start, *intending* that Reiki should flow to clear and cleanse your energy body. One of the easiest methods is the Reiki Shower technique.

THE REIKI SHOWER TECHNIQUE

This is a technique from the Japanese tradition, which is suitable for anyone with any level of Reiki. It consists of activating and cleansing your energy body (within your physical body and outside it throughout your aura) by absorbing Reiki energy throughout the body like a shower. You can use this technique almost anywhere for cleansing yourself, and it also helps to center yourself, raising your consciousness and bringing you into a pleasantly meditative state.

Stand or sit, and make yourself comfortable. Close or half close your eyes and begin to slow down and deepen your breathing until you can maintain a naturally slow and steady pace.

1. Place your hands in the Gassho position. This might more easily be described as a "prayer" position, with your palms together, fingers pointing upward, and

your hands held close to your body at the level of the heart chakra. Stay like this for a few moments, and intend to use Reiki to cleanse and activate your energy body.

2. Then separate your hands and lift them above your head, as high as possible, keeping them about 30–40 centimeters (12–15 inches) apart, with the palms facing each other. Wait for a few moments until you begin to feel the Reiki building up between your hands, and then turn your palms downward so that they are facing the top of your head.

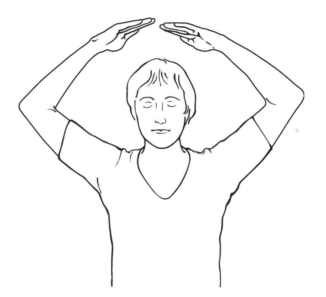

3. Visualize Reiki flowing out of your hands (as light, or like raindrops), and *intend* that you are receiving a shower of Reiki energy which flows over and through your whole physical and energy body, cleansing you and removing any negative energy. If you have Second

Degree, you can imagine an image of the power symbol flowing through you, and you can (silently) say its mantra three times, imagining it vibrating throughout your energy body.

4. When you feel the vibration of the Reiki energy flowing over and through you, move your hands, palms still facing toward you, and begin to draw them slowly down over your face and body, keeping your hands about 30–40 centimeters (12–15 inches) away from your body. *Intend* that Reiki is flowing from your hands, and continuing to cleanse and revitalize you as you draw your hands all the way down your body, and then down your legs to your feet, eventually turning your palms to face the floor and gently throwing the energy off your hands so that any negative energy flows out and into the earth below, to be healed and transformed.

5. Repeat this exercise a few times—I find three times to be ideal—and you should feel cleansed, revitalized and more alive as Reiki healing and light flow into all of your cells and fill every part of your body.

6. Place your hands together again in the Gassho position, spend a few moments experiencing gratitude for the Reiki and then finish. You may find it helpful to clap your hands once or twice, to help you to return to a more wakeful state if you feel a bit "spaced."

HATSUREI-HO

I think Hatsurei-ho (pronounced hat-soo-ray-hoe) is probably one of the most important of the original Japanese

Reiki techniques, as it is a way to enhance your Reiki channel and help you to grow spiritually. It can become a regular part of your spiritual practice, and is an ideal way to start the day, or to begin your practice of Reiki, whether treating yourself or other people, and is also an excellent way to end the day, just before sleep. The technique can take as little as ten minutes, or you can stretch out the more meditative parts of it (Joshin Kokyu Ho, the Cleansing Breath, and Seishin Toitsu, Concentration or Meditation) to half an hour or more—it's up to you.

The technique's basic functions are firstly to cleanse the outer part of your energy body (the aura) with dry bathing or brushing, then to cleanse the inner part of your energy body with the cleansing breath, and finally, when you are cleansed internally and externally, it allows you to bring more Reiki into yourself for your own personal healing, and to send Reiki out for global healing.

Kihon Shisei—Standard Posture

First make yourself comfortable, sitting either on the floor or on a chair, and then allow yourself to relax and close your eyes. Focus your attention on your hara point (Tan-den), which is 3–5 centimeters (1–2 inches) below your navel, and with your hands on your lap, palms facing downward, spend a few moments concentrating on bringing your breath into a slow, steady rhythm as you center yourself and focus your thoughts and *intend* to begin the Hatsurei-ho.

Kenyoku—Dry Bathing or Brushing Off

Now bring your focus to your breath. You should breathe out as you brush, making some sound when you exhale—e.g., a noisy, vigorous, sharp "Haaaaah." The brushing can be done either with contact, touching the body, or more easily without contact, about 5 centimeters (2 inches) away from your body, in the aura, and each of the movements (six in all) is completed quite quickly and positively.

Place the fingers of your right hand near the top of your left shoulder at the point where your collarbone meets your shoulder, fingers and thumb close together.

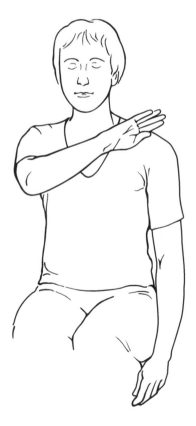

1. Draw your hand down quickly and positively diagonally across your chest in a straight line, down to your right hip. At the same time, expel your breath quickly and loudly throughout the movement—e.g., "Haaah."

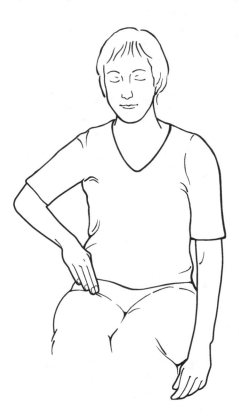

2. Now do the same thing on the other side, placing your left hand on your right shoulder, fingertips by the collarbone, and brush down from the right shoulder to the left hip, again exhaling loudly.
3. Return to your right hand on your left shoulder and repeat the process again, with your right hand brushing diagonally from your left shoulder to your right

hip and exhaling loudly. Next you are going to repeat the process, but this time, instead of brushing diagonally across your body, you will be brushing along your arms from shoulder to fingertips.

4. Place your right hand on the edge of your left shoulder, with your fingertips just on the edge of the shoulder, pointing slightly outward.

5. Keep your left arm straight and at your side, and draw your right hand quickly and positively down the outside of your arm, all the way to the fingertips of your left hand. At the same time, expel your breath quickly and loudly as before, making a definite sound throughout the movement.

6. Repeat this process on the other side, with your left hand on your right shoulder, brushing down quickly and positively to the fingertips of your right hand, expelling your breath loudly as before.

7. Complete this process by once more sweeping your right hand down your left arm from shoulder to fingertips, again exhaling loudly.

You will notice that each time the left side is brushed twice, while the right side is brushed only once. It has taken me some time to find out why, and I assumed it might be linked with three being a sacred number, but the most likely reason is apparently that in Japan the word for the number four is also the word for death, so they try to avoid repeating activities four times, or having four people around a table, etc., as it is considered unlucky. This habit is now so ingrained in Japanese culture that the Japanese scholar who told me about this said that they probably don't even realize why they are doing it.

Connect to Reiki

Now raise both your hands high up in the air above your head, with your palms facing each other about 30–40 centimeters (12–15 inches) apart, and visualize and feel the light and vibration of Reiki flowing into and between your hands and running through your whole body.

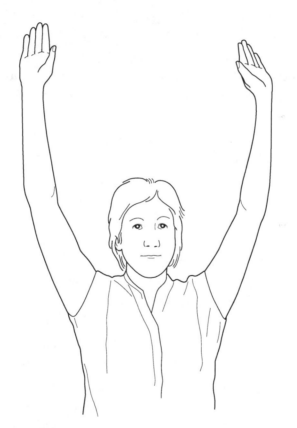

Joshin Kokyu Ho—the Cleansing Breath

1. Now lower your arms and put your hands on your lap with your palms facing upward, and let yourself

breathe naturally and steadily through your nose. Begin to focus your attention on your hara line—an energy line running through the center of your body, connecting all the major chakras from the crown down to the perineum—and allow your body to relax.

2. Concentrate on your breathing, and as you breathe in, visualize Reiki as white light pouring into you through your crown chakra, into your Reiki channel and down the hara line, and through your major chakras, and *intend* that the Reiki flows through you to cleanse away negativity and break through any blockages. Then imagine the Reiki spreading out, expanding to fill the whole of your body, from your head to your toes and from your shoulders to your fingertips, and sense it picking up any negativity and melting all your tensions away.

3. Next, as you breathe in even more Reiki, imagine it spreading out beyond your physical body into each of the seven layers of your aura, and sense the Reiki breaking through any blockages and picking up any negativity from your energy field.

4. Then each time you breathe out, *intend* to breathe out Reiki, and *intend* that the Reiki takes with it any negativity or blockages, out beyond your aura, where they can be healed and transformed by the Reiki.

5. Continue this process for a few minutes, or as long as you wish, breathing in Reiki to cleanse you, and breathing out Reiki so that it takes away any negativity.

6. Finally, take a really deep breath, blow out the rest of the negativity and then move on to the next section.

Gassho

When you feel ready, put your hands together in the Gassho (prayer) position and hold them in front of the center of your chest, at about the level of your heart chakra.

Seishin Toitsu—Concentration or Meditation

1. Keeping your hands in the Gassho position in front of your chest, take your focus away from breathing through your nose, and imagine that you are breathing through your hands.

2. As you breathe in, visualize the light of Reiki flowing in through your hands, and from there directly into your heart chakra. Imagine it filling your heart chakra and then sense it flowing into your hara line. Visualize it flowing up and down your hara line, so that your hara line is filled with light.

3. Next, as you breathe out, visualize that the Reiki light which now fills your hara line is spreading out to fill your whole body with healing energy, and then allow it to expand even further so that it flows through your skin, spreading out to fill your aura, healing your whole energy field.

4. Then imagine it flowing beyond your aura in all directions to infinity, radiating out through your hands, flowing out and spreading Reiki in all directions, expanding its healing, balancing, harmonizing energy wherever it is needed—to people, animals, birds, fish and other creatures, to trees and other plants, and to the planet itself.

5. Continue this process for as long as you wish, and let your mind settle into a peaceful, meditative state.

Gokai Sansho

In the traditional way, Japanese Reiki students would at this point say the Reiki principles aloud three times—obviously in Japanese! You may feel you would like to do the same, either in Japanese or in English.

Japanese	English
Kyo dake wa (*Kee oh dah kay wah*)	Just for today
Okoru-na (*Oh koh roo nah*)	Do not get angry
Shinpai suna (*Shin pie soo nah*)	Do not worry
Kansha shite (*Kan shah she tay*)	Show appreciation (or be grateful)
Goo hage me (*Gyo oh hah gay may*)	Work hard (on yourself)
Hito ni shinsetsu ni (*Hee toe nee shin set soo nee*)	Be kind to others

Mokunen

Place your hands back onto your lap with palms facing downward, and intend that the Hatsurei-ho be completed. When you feel ready, open your eyes and shake your hands gently for a few seconds, to bring you back to a greater state of physical awareness.

You are now ready to get on with your day, or to begin your practice of Reiki either as a self-treatment, or the treatment of others.

OTHER TECHNIQUES FOR PERSONAL ENERGETIC CLEANSING

Cold Showers

Yes, I know this might be an unpleasant thought, but to cleanse both your physical and energy bodies fully I recommend a cold shower—this is an essential part of many Eastern spiritual traditions. If you have any health condition that might make you particularly susceptible to shock from the cold water, ask your doctor before adding this technique to your cleansing routine.

Cold water is different energetically from hot water, and when its vital cleansing energy flows over your physical body and through your energy field, the "shock" of it shakes loose the negative or "sticky" energy that is trapped in and around your body. Of course, a warm or hot shower or bath is how most of us prefer to clean our physical bodies, and they can also be very relaxing, but energetically they have the effect of expanding your aura, which can potentially make the negative, "sticky" energy enter further into your energy body so it becomes harder to remove. That is why it is important to *start* your shower with cold water rather than ending with it, although you can do *both* if you wish.

However, I'm not asking you to be a masochist and stand under the showerhead for ages, although in other traditions, such as Kundalini yoga, a 20- or 30-minute cold shower is recommended. I am only suggesting that you let the cold water flow over your chakras and main meridian points, so that they are cleansed, and this can be done quite quickly and easily. The whole process needs to take no more than 15 to 20 seconds. If you wish, you can quickly jump under the cold water, and turn around so that the water flows over the crown of your head, and down all the front and back chakras, as well as the minor chakras and main meridian points on your shoulders, elbows, wrists, hands, hips, knees, ankles and feet, and then turn the water temperature up to what you normally prefer. (You can wear a shower cap unless you want to wash your hair, as your crown chakra will still be cleansed by the water flowing over the cap.)

If you don't have a shower at home, it is possible to buy shower attachments that fit onto most bath taps, or you can use a jug instead. Just fill it with cold water, and pour it over your chakras. Afterward, you can fill the jug with comfortably hot water, and use it to warm yourself up (or fill the bath instead), although a vigorous toweling or wrapping yourself in a terry robe will do the job, too.

For most people, I recommend at least two cold showers a day: one first thing in the morning, to wash off any negative energies generated during the night, and then another one before bed, to wash off the negative "stuff" we pick up during an average day. However, if you work in any of the caring professions, or as a therapist or counselor, or doing any other work where you are frequently dealing with negative people, I would really recommend a cold shower as soon as you get in from work, which will get rid of any "psychic pollution" you have picked up during the day, and help you to feel refreshed and ready to enjoy your evening.

Using Reiki in Your Usual Cleansing Routine

In addition to cold showers, you can use Reiki to enhance the effects of your usual cleansing routine. When holding the showerhead in your hand, you can *intend* that Reiki flows out of your hand into the water, to cleanse and heal you as you shower, or if you have Second Degree, you can draw a power symbol over your showerhead before you begin. You can also draw the power symbol over your bath water, before you step in (or when you are sitting in it, if you forget), or if you don't know the symbols, simply *intend* that Reiki flows from your hands into your bath water, so that you are bathing in cleansing, healing water. Add a few drops of lavender oil, light some candles, and you have the perfect remedial, relaxing retreat. (But remember not to leave a burning candle unattended.)

TECHNIQUES FOR CLEANSING YOUR ENVIRONMENT

Where Do You Need to Cleanse?

Because you can potentially pick up negative energies anywhere, the answer should probably be "everywhere," but obviously that isn't practical. Basically, you need to regularly clean and cleanse all the areas in which you spend any substantial amount of time, and for most people that means their home and their workplace, or at least their immediate surroundings at their place of work. At home, the areas you need to concentrate on are the corners of each room, where negative or stagnant energy can collect, and places where you sit often, and especially where you sleep, so your bed and favorite chair are important. You can use Reiki to clear, harmonize and protect any spaces you occupy, and the most effective way is to place power symbols in each corner of each room, and on the floor and ceiling, and also on any furniture where you spend lots of time, such as your bed or favorite chair, and imagine and *intend* that the whole room be filled with Reiki. However, if you don't have Second Degree, you can still use Reiki for cleansing by just sitting quietly and visualizing and *intending* that Reiki flows from your palms to fill the whole room with healing energy and light, perhaps imagining the light of Reiki flowing like a soft mist until it fills the whole space.

If you spend any time in areas where there are lots of people, especially paved areas such as city streets, shopping centers or supermarkets, or in other potentially negative places like hospitals or funeral parlors, you might pick up negative energy, especially on your shoes. Such places can have a layer of "sticky" negative energy lying around at ground level, so you are virtually wading through a "soup" of negative energy which can attach itself to your shoes, so it makes sense to take them off by the door—or at least to walk on a patch of natural ground, such as grass—before you walk into your home.

It is also a good idea to take on some of the principles of feng shui by clearing out any clutter in your home, and then keeping it clean and tidy. You may think I'm rather boring to be encouraging you to carry out more housework—I don't like it much either—but you'll be surprised by how much better your environment "feels" when it is clean as well as energetically clear, and that applies equally to your work environment and your home.

chapter twelve

PERSONAL GROWTH AND SPIRITUAL DEVELOPMENT

Reiki is more than just a healing therapy for physical problems; it is a tool for personal growth and spiritual development, because it works holistically, healing and balancing our emotional and psychological states, and promoting self-knowledge. In many spiritual traditions it is necessary to study and meditate for many years to reach an understanding of the meaning of your own life, but Reiki begins to awaken your sense of the divine that exists within everyone and everything, right from the first time you begin to use it. The very act of treating yourself every day with Reiki is itself a spiritual discipline; the meditative quality of self-treatment encourages a sense of peace and tranquility, and a feeling of oneness with everything around you. At a certain stage in your development in Reiki this may manifest as a need to live your life in a spiritual way (which is as individual as the person—there is no "right" or "wrong" way to live spiritually). As the Reiki continues to flow through you, you continue to grow and develop as a unique human being.

THE REIKI PRINCIPLES

One of the primary tools for personal growth and spiritual development is the integration of the five Reiki principles into your life. The traditional history tells that Dr. Usui received inspiration during meditation about the healing of the spirit through a conscious decision to take responsibility for one's own health and well-being, in order for the Reiki healing energies to have lasting results. He also gained insight into the way people will take for granted, or not value, those things that they receive too freely and easily. It is said that he was then given the five spiritual principles of Reiki that would balance the physical healing. However, we now know from research into the Japanese origins of Reiki that the five principles of Reiki adopted by Dr. Usui were originally suggested as guidelines for a fulfilled life by the Meiji emperor of Japan, inspired by ancient Buddhist precepts.

There are several variations of these five Reiki principles, and some of these have been given in earlier chapters, including the translation of the original written by Usui (see page 27). My favorite interpretation, which I believe follows the essence of his teachings, is as follows:

Just for today, I will let go of anger;
Just for today, I will let go of worry;
Just for today, I will give thanks for my many blessings;
Just for today, I will do my work diligently;
Just for today, I will be kind to every living creature.

Living in the Present

Possibly one of the most important aspects of the above principles is the phrase "Just for today." Living in the moment, focusing on the present, being aware of what is going on around you, forces you to live in the *now*. And the *now* is the time you are actually living, the only moment over which you have any control, the moment of power. But most of us spend much of each day thinking about the past or the futures. For example:

Past Feeling angry, guilty, regretful or nostalgic about what we did an hour ago, yesterday, last week or last year.

Future Feeling worried, hopeful, excited or apprehensive about what we're planning to do tonight, tomorrow, next week or next month.

Ask yourself honestly what thoughts have been flitting through your mind even while you've been reading this book. Are they anything like these?

- "What shall we have for tea tonight?"
- "I wonder if I locked the car?"
- "Did I put those papers I need in the trash by mistake?"
- "What time am I supposed to be at . . . ?"

Or perhaps you've been going through an inventory of imperatives such as: "I must . . . ;" "I should . . . ;" "I ought to . . . ;" "Why didn't I . . . ?" or you have a whole host of "what if" scenarios on your mind, such as "What if I lose my job?" or "What if I can't pay that bill?" or "What if I get ill, how will I cope?"

The past is gone, and the future hasn't arrived yet, so why not really notice and enjoy whatever it is you are doing right now? And if you're not enjoying it, then do something else! Living in the present is so much more rewarding than constantly thinking about the past or the future. You can begin to really feel, really see, and really hear what is going on around you. When did you last *really* see the color of a flower, feel the texture of a velvety petal, linger on the delicious scent? Can you even envisage doing that right now?

ACTIVITY — LIVING IN THE MOMENT

Try this awareness-raising exercise for a few minutes, to fully utilize your senses to pick up all the sensations of the present moment.

◆ Find a comfortable place to sit, and spend a few moments settling down, perhaps by deepening and slowing your breathing, until you feel quite relaxed. Then close your eyes and focus your attention on what you can hear around you. Really listen. What are the sounds? Birds singing, nearby traffic, a radio in the next room, a dog barking, a clock ticking, people's voices? Let your awareness spread out, and see if you can hear even more.

◆ Now turn your attention to what you can smell. Breathe in the air slowly, letting the smells linger in your nostrils. What can you smell? The fragrance of fresh flowers, perfume or room freshener, or the smell of stale tobacco or sweaty clothes? Are there any food smells, perhaps baking bread or the aroma of fresh coffee? Open your mouth to let the air flow over your taste buds, and see if you can expand your sense of smell to pick up even more odors from what is around you.

◆ Next, pay attention to your sense of touch. Are you aware of different parts of your body, or its weight in the chair? Can you feel the texture of your clothes against your skin, or the warmth of the sun or the softness of a breeze against your face? Feel your body moving as you breathe in and out, and perhaps tense the muscles in your shoulders and then let them relax, feeling the different sensations as they change.

◆ Now open your eyes and let yourself look around you. Really look. Notice the light and shade, the colors and shapes, the patterns and designs. Pick out one color, and notice the different shades and tones of that color, from deep and dark to pale and light. If there is a plant nearby, examine the structure of its leaves, the way they join the main stem, the delicate formation of buds about to burst into new growth. Look down at your own hands, and see the texture and color of the skin, the wrinkles around the knuckles, the smoothness of the nails. Turn your palms upward and notice the myriad lines, some deep, some light and fine.

Notice the shape of your palm, and the different lengths of your fingers. Have you ever paid this much attention to any part of your body before?

♦ Now spend a few moments integrating this experience. This is what your life is like at this moment in time. For a few minutes you have really paid attention to what is going on around you, to what you are doing. How does that feel? Have you ever felt this "awake" to your surroundings before? This is truly living in the present.

♦ Just allow yourself a few moments to "come around" from this heightened state of awareness, and then continue with whatever you had planned to do. Obviously it would be difficult to maintain such a state of awareness all the time—you simply couldn't concentrate on anything else and your brain's interpretation of your senses would rapidly become overloaded. However, do try this exercise occasionally to remind yourself of the sheer magic of living in a human body that gives us all these amazing sensations which we so readily take for granted.

Now to return to the five Reiki principles, I'd like to encourage you to explore them in more depth.

Just for Today, I Will Let Go of Anger

Anger is such a destructive emotion, and often we express our anger to the people we care about the most, so it hurts us as much as it hurts them. Anger is usually tied to expectations about what you believe should or should not be happening, or to responses about things that have happened in the past. But believe it or not, anger is a conscious choice, and is often just a habit. You've probably been reacting in a similar way in similar circumstances for years, but you *can* choose not to be angry—just for today.

Of course I'm not saying that you should never experience anger—that would be unrealistic. However, anger is only one of a whole range of responses at your disposal, any of which might gain you a better result, and which you could choose to use instead—but first you have to take a deep breath and let go of that habitual response. Perhaps that old adage to count to ten before speaking isn't so silly, after all.

Think of a situation in which you usually get angry. When a teenage son or daughter gets home late? Or when your partner forgets your birthday? When someone at work makes a mistake that will take you days to sort out? Or when a neighbor cuts the hedge and all the clippings fall into your garden? In each of these cases anger is only one way to respond to the situation. At such times we often put blame on the other person, saying, "You made me angry by . . ." but the reality is that you chose to be angry. Other people can't make you feel emotions. Certainly, other people's actions can cause you to react, but the type of reaction is up to you.

The most obvious way in which you could change the tone of the situation would be to talk about it calmly and rationally, expressing your feelings in a way that doesn't hurt the other person. With the teenager, you could explain not only that you were worried but also why you were worried. To your partner you could explain that you feel hurt, and why being forgotten about means you feel that way. In the case of your work colleague, maybe you need to find out why they made such a mistake—had they been trained properly, or shown exactly what was needed? And surely it would be reasonable to get them to help to put things right? In the case of your neighbor's transgression into your space, maybe you just need to bite the bullet and realize that some hedge clippings are bound to fall your way, so look upon it as a bonus for your compost heap!

It's all about adopting a different approach, and communicating properly and sensibly. It's also about making a conscious choice to let go, to embrace an attitude of forgiveness, understanding and conciliation, rather than anger, misunderstanding, blaming and confrontation. To let go of anger is to release what is blocking you from giving and receiving unconditional love. Perhaps it sounds like an oversimplification, but try it—just for today. It really works.

Just for Today, I Will Let Go of Worry

Living in the present can be so much more comfortable, because you really can choose not to worry. Worry is our usual response to a probable event in the future, to a "what if" scenario, to something that might occur, but which nine times out of ten doesn't. Our tendency is to put ourselves through hell in our minds, contemplating what could come to pass, yet if we look at the present moment, which is all we really have, there is no great problem at all.

Worrying can be another habit we get into, so just for a moment think about some situations where you would normally worry. Going to the dentist? Taking a test? Attending an interview for a new job? Not having enough money to pay the bills? Apart from the last one, all of the above are "one-off" situations that usually last only for a short time. A visit to the dentist might take as little as ten minutes, but I know people who can put themselves through three weeks of agony while waiting for the event. If you're taking a test or attending an interview, worrying isn't going to give you a better chance, but study and planning will. And in the case of not having enough money, worrying isn't going to help, either. If there's some action you can take, like writing to creditors, visiting the bank manager, asking the utility provider for more time to pay, or getting advice from the Citizens Advice Bureau, then do it. If there's nothing you can do, then just let go.

I'm a firm believer that while we struggle and strive to control a situation, we're just creating an energy cycle that makes things worse, whereas when we let go and stop worrying about the situation, something good comes along to sort it out. That "good" may be a person, some useful advice or just the right amount of money, but it's amazing how often just the right thing turns up.

In essence, then, worry is a wasted emotion. If you can do something about your problem, do it, and if you can't do anything, stop worrying about it, because no one has ever changed any situation just by worrying—all it does is make you feel awful. However, as a last resort, and if you're really determined to worry, choose an appropriate time, make yourself a cup of tea or pour yourself a drink, and give yourself half an hour to have a really good worry—then you can forget about it for the rest of the week! Yes, I know that's a silly suggestion, but maybe its very silliness puts worry into perspective, because worrying is extremely unhelpful and inappropriate for someone who lives in the moment, so you can choose not to worry—just for today.

Just for Today, I Will Give Thanks for My Many Blessings

This is sometimes shown as "honor our parents, teachers and elders," and for years I thought I understood this. Indeed, as I had been brought up to be polite I assumed I was already fulfilling this dictate. However, I eventually came to understand that its influence is much wider. It really means that we should honor and be grateful to everyone: to partners, friends, neighbors, colleagues, children, shop assistants, bus drivers, receptionists, farmers, chefs—in fact, every person we meet, under any circumstances. Every interaction with another person is a potential learning experience. The shop assistants gossiping about last night's party instead of serving you are teaching you patience. The gang of teenage boys shouting obscenities in the street is teaching you tolerance. The girl with an amputated leg is teaching you compassion. The tiny baby you hold in your arms is teaching you love.

All the time we are making conscious choices when we make contact with people, choosing those from whom we wish to learn, those we want as friends, those we need to work with. My personal belief (and I recognize that for some people this might prove very challenging, so feel free to reject it if it is upsetting) is that as a soul we even choose our parents, before we are born, for the value of the experiences we will gain from them—whether those experiences are good or bad. So we need to honor and respect all the people in our lives, because we have chosen them to help us to incarnate and grow spiritually.

But even wider than that, the ideal that we should be grateful for our many blessings means that we have to recognize those blessings first—and often, we don't. If life is difficult, if we're going through a "bad patch," we tend to see things from a very morose perspective, and to assume that everything in life is bad. Even when life is relatively calm and happy we are often not aware of it, and take it very much for granted. Yet most of us are living very good lives, even if they aren't perfect.

Take a good, hard look at your life for a few minutes. I hope and expect that you have a reasonably warm and comfortable home, enough clothes and a good selection of foods to eat. You probably have much more than just these basics. You may have a loving family around you, a faithful dog to go walking with and lots of friends with whom to socialize. Materially you might have lots of "things," from a washing machine, a microwave oven or a CD player, to beautiful jewelry, a golf-club membership or a sports car. Even if you don't have many—or any—of those things, there are still bound to be lots of things in your life worth being grateful for, from the beauty of a sunset to the warmth of an open fire; from the gentle touch of a lover to the sweet kiss of a small child. Why not get a large piece of paper and list all the good things in your life, from the simple to the extravagant? I'm sure you'll be amazed at how many there are.

I believe it is important to develop an "attitude of gratitude," to constantly remind ourselves of the wonderful world we live in and to remember to enjoy it. Take time out of every day just to stand and stare, whether at the beauty of a flower or at a happy child at play, it doesn't matter. What matters is that we develop an awareness of life, and what it means to live it. Of course there will be ups and downs, and sometimes we'll be happy and sometimes we'll be sad, but every experience is valuable because it helps to make us who we are. So, just for today, give thanks for your many blessings.

Just for Today, I Will Do My Work Diligently

Work in this sense is not simply earning a living. It is all types of work, from everyday tasks like cooking a meal for ourselves or our families, to working on our self-development through meditation or reading inspirational books. We often confuse what we do with who we are, taking our sense of identity from the kind of job we do—or don't do. This is one of the major reasons why being labeled as "unemployed" can be so stressful, because if we only recognize ourselves for our job title, being without a job takes away our sense of self.

What we need to remember is that we are human *beings*, not human *doings*! We are *all* valuable and special; every life, every person, has a role to play in the whole— we all impact on each other in so many ways.

It is important to respect any "job" that we have chosen for ourselves, and honor ourselves by doing our best to create a feeling of satisfaction in that work—that is working "diligently." *All* work is valuable to the extent that we choose to value it, so value yourself whatever work you do, in the home, at school or college, as a voluntary worker or in some place of employment. Take satisfaction from even the simplest tasks. There is another well-known quotation: "Before enlightenment, chop wood, carry water; after enlightenment, chop wood, carry water." No matter how spiritual your life may become, no matter how many hours a day you spend in meditation, no matter how many spiritually uplifting books you read—even if you become a monk or a nun—you will still need to work to feed yourself, to clothe yourself, to keep yourself warm, to live comfortably. It is probably true that there may be some jobs that, if you have such a choice, you might wish to avoid, and others that, as you grow personally and spiritually, will be more attractive to you. But being in the present means enjoying and valuing what you are doing right now. It means doing everything to the best of your ability. So, just for today, do your work diligently.

Just for Today, I Will Be Kind to Every Living Creature

As your consciousness is raised with Reiki, you know instinctively that every living thing is a part of you, and you are a part of it, and that everything is a part of the divine, God, the Source or whatever you choose to call it. It therefore becomes natural to treat everyone and everything with kindness and respect. We come to realize that there is no place for prejudice, judgmentalism, cruelty or indifference in a world where we are all connected and a part of the whole. All people, animals, birds, fish, reptiles, insects and plants have a vital role to play, and should therefore be valued and respected.

With this connectedness in mind, if we are not kind to someone else, we are not being loving and respecting of ourselves, so actually the caring needs to start with ourselves. How kind are you to yourself? Do you always put other people's needs before your own? Do you forgive yourself when you make mistakes, or do you endlessly "beat yourself up" over them? Do you give yourself regular "treats" to make yourself feel good? Do these questions make you feel a bit uncomfortable?

The trouble is that most of us are not brought up to feel good about ourselves, let alone to be kind to ourselves. In Britain, and some other Western cultures, it is seen as being "good" to be modest, polite and unemotional (all those stiff upper lips!), and to "keep yourself to yourself." No wonder we find it so hard to accept praise, say what we feel, cry when we're sad, hug each other, admit when we're lonely . . . or, heaven forbid, actually say good things about ourselves. We seem to have so many unwritten rules about our behavior that other cultures don't have. Other nationalities can be more open and more exuberant, and can enjoy life more, without being censured.

So why not try a little experiment? Imagine that instead of behaving in a typically "British," or even "North American" way, you come from a warm Mediterranean or South American country. Hug and kiss your relatives and friends. Laugh—or cry—whenever you feel like it. Tell everyone you meet how great they look. Smile at complete strangers. Buy yourself a little present—just because you are you, and you want to celebrate the fact. That is what it is like to be kind to yourself—to express the real you in the world.

The more you practice being thoughtful and loving, the easier it gets, and it rubs off on the way you react to everyone around you. Kindness then becomes a habit. Try committing some "random acts of kindness and senseless acts of beauty." Give the parking attendant the money to pay for the next car, as well as for your own; buy a bunch of flowers for a friend when it's not their birthday; offer to weed the garden for an elderly neighbor you don't know very well; take a box of chocolates to a nearby nursing home, even when you know no one there; compliment someone in the bus line on their perfume. Little things like these can make other people feel good, and doing them will make you feel good. And of course, there's a saying "what goes around, comes around," so as you do good things for others, nice things will happen to you, too.

So, just for today, value yourself for the important difference you make to the universe; treat yourself with the respect you would give to a special friend; and be kind to every person you interact with and to every living thing you encounter.

ACTIVITY—AFFIRMATIONS USING THE REIKI PRINCIPLES

The Reiki principles are a really good code of ethics to live by, but you can bring them into your life in a very active way by turning them into affirmations. If you have particular problems letting go of anger or worry, for example, then put those principles firmly into the present tense, so that they become:

- Today, I let go of anger.
- Today, I let go of worry.
- Today, I am grateful for my many blessings.
- Today, I am working diligently.
- Today, I am kind to everyone and everything around me.

You can make them even more positive by expanding them like this:

- Today, I let go of anger, allowing peace and tranquility to flow into my life.
- Today, I let go of worry, accepting easily and happily the natural flow of my life.
- Today, I am grateful for the many blessings that make my life so rich and full.
- Today, I am working diligently on my personal and spiritual development, and on any tasks I am required to carry out.
- Today, I value, respect and show kindness to everyone and everything around me.

Then say the affirmations out loud at least 20 times a day, and they can be even more effective if you do this while looking at yourself in a mirror. Okay, it might make you feel slightly uncomfortable, perhaps, but the effect tends to be more immediate. While you are saying the affirmations you may get a reaction, such as your inner voice saying, "I can't do that" or even, "I won't do that." If so, just acknowledge it, let it go, and carry on with the affirmation. Eventually the resistance will fade, and you will begin to feel that it is easier to let go of these difficult emotions.

You can carry on with the affirmations for as long as you wish, but use your intuition and when you feel the time is right, stop saying them. To test whether using the affirmations has helped after a week or so, you might like to try drawing up a list of things that make you angry or worried. You may be surprised at how difficult it is to think of things to put on the list!

DOES REIKI CONFLICT WITH ANY RELIGION?

If we are looking at Reiki for spiritual development, we need also to look at it in relation to religion. To consider Reiki historically, it is an energy science that predates the Christian or Islamic faiths—it originates from Buddhist practices from around 500 years before Christ was born, and about 1,000 years before Mohammed. However, the system of Reiki we use in the West, based on the teachings of Mikao Usui, is not a belief system, and is not in conflict with Christian, Muslim or other religious beliefs. Indeed, Usui is believed to have met and engaged in discussions with a number of Christians, and many of his students, and some of the Masters he trained, were Christians. Perhaps most important, one of those Christians was Dr. Chujiro Hayashi, who clearly did not consider Reiki to be contradictory to his beliefs. Western

Reiki's lineage is through Dr. Hayashi, who taught Hawayo Takata, who taught the 22 Masters through whom Reiki has spread throughout the Western world since the mid-1970s.

Surely the main point here is "that which is good is from God"? We are told in the Bible that Jesus laid his hands on people to heal them (John 14:12; Matthew 10:8), but the laying on of hands for healing has been a part of many cultures and many religions for millennia. Of course, throughout history the Christian faith (and other religions, too) has feared and distrusted mystical knowledge—that is, an awareness of things it could not understand—but surely being spiritual should be less about religion and more about behavior? And surely this should include being tolerant of things that we don't necessarily understand?

Reiki is a safe, nonintrusive complementary health-care modality with no known contraindications, which many people find to be a helpful support for their health and well-being, whether they are using it themselves, or receiving it from practitioners.

Some Reiki practitioners may have rather unconventional views, it is true, but belief in Reiki guides, channeling and so on, somewhat unkindly called "flaky Reiki," are new aspects of modern Reiki styles—they were not part of Usui's original Reiki system as it was first taught in the West. But Reiki is practiced by people of many different faiths all over the world, and just because someone has a different belief system from your own does not make them a "bad" person, or the health care practice they offer something "evil." There is a beauty and peace in the practice of Reiki that can fit easily into anyone's spiritual life. Despite the emphasis on words such as "spiritual" and "soul," Reiki is not seen in the West as a religion, although in Japan it is considered more as a spiritual practice. Even its roots in Buddhism do not really constitute a religion, as Buddhism is a way of life, so it does not conflict with or pose any threat to those with specific beliefs. What we try to promote within the practice of Reiki is an environment of tolerance and acceptance, so we do not judge our students or clients by their religious beliefs. We would wish that others would behave in the same way toward us.

chapter thirteen

BEING CREATIVE WITH REIKI

Throughout this book I have stressed that the potential with Reiki is unlimited, so it isn't just for your own self-healing, or for the healing of other people. It can be used creatively in lots of different ways—the only limitation is your own imagination. The aim of this chapter is to suggest various ways in which you might use Reiki, but hopefully these suggestions will spark off even more of your own ideas. I would just like to encourage you to use Reiki as much as possible to foster healing, harmony and balance in the world around you. Have fun!

CREATIVE IDEAS FOR USING REIKI WITH PEOPLE

Sending Reiki Through the Aura

There are times when it isn't possible to treat someone by laying your hands on them, for instance at the scene of an accident, or to soothe a crying child or an agitated animal, and in these cases it is perfectly acceptable to send the Reiki through the aura. Just imagine your aura expanding until it encompasses the person or animal to whom you wish the Reiki to flow, and then mentally "switch on" the Reiki by *intending* that it should flow. If you wish, you can hold your hands out in the general direction of the recipient, although this isn't strictly necessary, and may look a bit odd under certain circumstances. If the person or animal is accepting of the Reiki, you will start to feel it flowing from your hands; if not, then nothing will happen—and if so, don't judge that person or animal for not wishing to receive healing, for whatever reason. Each of us is on our own individual journey through life, and we cannot know why Reiki might not be appropriate at that particular time.

Distant/Absent Reiki

As mentioned in Chapter 7, to carry out really efficient distant healing with Reiki you need the techniques that are taught at Second Degree level, which enable you to send very powerful healing to anyone, anywhere, at any time (including the past and the future) using the symbols taught at that level. These techniques also allow you to carry out a complete Reiki treatment on someone at a distance, with exactly the same effectiveness as if they were receiving a hands-on treatment, which is often a stunning experience, both for the person sending the Reiki and the recipient.

However, don't be put off if you haven't done Reiki 2 yet—it is possible to send some healing at First Degree level, although it is unlikely to be quite as strong. As a simile, I usually describe distance healing at Second Degree level as like a laser beam, where there is no diminution of strength regardless of distance, whereas at First Degree it is more like a normal flashlight beam that spreads out and loses light the further it goes. If you want to send healing and love to people, just write their names on a piece of paper and hold the paper in your hands, *intending* that Reiki should go to them. You can use a photograph in the same way, holding it in your hands and focusing your thoughts on that person, *intending* that Reiki should flow to them for their highest and greatest good, which should not be limited only to the individual person, but to others around them who might be affected, too.

Using Reiki on Personal Problems and Situations

Whatever kinds of problems you are having, from strained relationships with your partner or family, to difficulties at work or with studying, you can use Reiki to help to permeate the situation with healing. Simply write the situation down on paper—whether it needs a single sentence or several paragraphs—and then hold the paper between your hands, *intending* that Reiki should flow to the situation for the highest and greatest good of all. (Which means, of course, that you cannot control anyone else using this method—it is not ethical to try to get someone you like to love you, or to wish a colleague you dislike would leave their job, and Reiki won't work for you in that way.)

You really need to give Reiki to the situation for at least ten minutes a day for as long as the situation exists, and you also need to detach yourself from specific expectations about the result. This can be difficult, because it is human to want a particular result. However, Reiki always works for the highest good, and although we might believe we know what is best for us, we are not always right. You have to trust Reiki to bring you what you *need*, even if that isn't necessarily what you want. Again, there are techniques taught at Second Degree level which make working on problems and situations even more effective—draw the distant symbol over the paper first, to connect with the situation, then the harmony symbol to bring harmony to the situation, and finally the power symbol, to bring Reiki powerfully into the situation.

Empowering Affirmations and Goals

You can use a similar method for working on your goals and dreams with Reiki. Write down what you really want—a new job, a loving relationship (but not naming a particular person), a cottage in the country, a trip to Disneyland—on a piece of paper, and be as specific as possible. Write down all the aspects of what you are seeking, so if you want a cottage in the country, put down how many bedrooms and bathrooms you want, what kind of kitchen, whether you want central heating or open fires, a small garden or acres of farmland, etc. Then hold the piece of paper in your hands and give it Reiki for at least ten minutes a day until you achieve what you want—or until your circumstances change and you realize it isn't any longer what you really desire.

But beware—be sure you really want something before you ask for it. (That's why you need to be very particular in how you describe it.) If it is for your highest and greatest good to receive what you've asked for, then Reiki will work with your Higher Self to achieve it—

but do remember that sometimes our highest and greatest good can be served by the changes we go through during difficult times, as well as in happy times. So if you do achieve what you've asked for, and it turns out to be less enjoyable than you expected, then try to accept that it is a lesson well learned, and move on.

If you are working with affirmations—positive statements that can help to reprogram your thinking—then these can be made even more effective by writing them down and holding the paper in your hands, saying them over and over to yourself while giving them Reiki. This can be a powerful method for change, so make sure that your affirmations are always really positive, and are fully in the present. So, for example, use "I have a wonderful, loving relationship with a man/woman who loves me" even if this isn't the case right at this moment in time, rather than "I will have . . ." If you use a statement founded in the future, such as "I will have," then it continues to be in the future, rather than potentially becoming a part of your reality now.

Using Color with Reiki

Light is part of the wide spectrum of energy that surrounds us, and the visible part of light (i.e., excluding such rays as infrared and ultraviolet) is split into the spectrum of colors we see in a rainbow. Colors can be a powerful force in healing because, whether you realize it or not, at a physical, mental and emotional level we respond to them. You can therefore enhance the effects of Reiki on certain situations by visualizing an appropriate colored light enfolding yourself, the person or animal you are treating, or a specific part of the body. Clearly, using the same color that vibrates to a particular chakra (see Chapter 4) will help with those points of the body, but in color healing it is customary to use eight colors, not just the seven we refer to in the rainbow.

Color / Theme	Effects
Red *Energy*	Red encourages vitality, sexuality, strength and willpower, so it is good to use if you lack mental or physical energy, or when you're tired and apathetic. On a physical level, it energizes the nervous system, stimulates the senses, activates the circulatory system, stimulates the kidneys, adrenals and reproductive organs, increases the pulse rate and inhalation rate and raises blood pressure, and is useful for healing infections.
Orange *Joy*	Orange encourages happiness, fun, joyfulness and pleasure, so use it to combat depression, lethargy and procrastination, to replace them with feelings of lightness and emotional release. Physically, orange encourages movement and dance, stimulates the thyroid and stomach, and helps to strengthen the lungs, bronchial tubes and bones.
Yellow *Detachment*	Yellow helps to increase objectivity and intellectual powers, so use it when you find it difficult to detach from people, possessions, ideas or situations, or when you can't make decisions. Physically, yellow stimulates the

lymphatic system, digestion, and the motor and sensory nerves, and encourages better hormone production, as well as stimulating overall body repair.

Green *Balance*

Green is cleansing, balancing and calming, so use it if your life is out of balance because of overwork, stress or worry. Physically, green can help you to bring more balance into your eating habits to encourage better health as it helps to balance the physical body and the cerebrum, stimulates the pituitary, and is reported to act as a germicide and to help combat tumors.

Turquoise
Immunity

Turquoise is cool, refreshing and soothing, so it is useful for calming nervousness, or for when you feel dominated by others—i.e., you lack immunity to their influence, so it encourages you to value your own thoughts and ideas. On a physical level, use turquoise to strengthen the immune system, counteract inflammation and fever, heal burned skin or repair acute problems.

Blue *Relaxation*

Blue is calming, relaxing and peaceful, so use it to combat tension, nervousness, insomnia, impatience and stressful situations such as a "workaholic" lifestyle when you're rushed, anxious and feel you have no time. Physically, blue acts as a sedative, so use it to relieve fevers, inflammations, itching or irritations, and to encourage good sleep patterns or cope with anxiety. It also stimulates the pineal gland and the parathyroid, and is said to be helpful in shrinking abscesses or tumors.

Violet *Dignity*

Violet is for dignity, reverence, prayer, meditation and purpose, so it encourages calmness and balance in body and mind. Use it if you need to work on feelings of self-worth and self-respect, as well as to increase respect for your home, work and other people, and to encourage feelings of inner beauty. On a physical level, violet activates the spleen and white blood cells, helps to reduce fevers and relax muscles, lowers body temperature, heart rate and blood pressure, and slows down the action of the kidneys and lungs.

Magenta
Letting Go

Magenta is said to be the color of spiritual fulfillment, so it induces contentment and feelings of completeness. Use it at times when you need to let go of old memories, thought patterns and unwanted emotions, leaving you free to change and grow. It can also be helpful when you want to make changes in your routines or lifestyle, in letting go of obsessions, negative thoughts and unhelpful habits. Physically, magenta helps to stimulate the kidneys and adrenals, balances emotions, and is said to help to adjust and balance blood pressure.

Reiki Groups

Getting together with other people who do Reiki is great fun, and the more confident and experienced members can help those who are new to Reiki, or who feel shy about trying it on their family or friends without getting some more practice first, so it gives them a chance to hone their skills in a friendly and nurturing environment. The more Reiki you receive, the more you heal, and the more Reiki energy will flow through you so that you can help others to heal, so Reiki groups are an ideal place to "swap" treatments with one another.

To have two, four, six or even more people treating you at once can be a delightful experience, producing an even deeper state of relaxation. (It doesn't have to be even numbers, but it is often easier that way.) Of course, the more people you have treating you, the less time it takes, as you simply share the hand positions between you, usually with each person working on one side of the body only. If you have lots of people you can cover all of the body and the legs, feet, arms and hands as well—and of course everyone can take turns receiving Reiki, as well as giving it.

When treating in a large group, don't feel too constrained by the traditional hand positions. It is often more comfortable to spread out a little. For example, with the head positions it would be silly for four people to be crowded so close together, all trying to treat the head at the same time, so it is better to have one person with both their hands underneath the recipient's head, and then one on either side with one hand by the person's ear and the other hand by their neck. This would mean the eyes would not be treated—but with three people treating the head area there would definitely be enough Reiki to go around! Other people can be spaced out on either side, treating the body and the legs, and another person could be at the end of the table, treating the person's feet.

If you like this idea, why not start a Reiki group yourself? You could contact the people who trained on the same course as you, or any other Reiki people you know. Alternatively, various Reiki organizations have lists of Reiki groups, so you could join with one of those (see Resources, page 281, for some contact details).

OTHER CREATIVE WAYS OF USING REIKI

Using Reiki with Food and Drink

It makes good sense to give Reiki to all the food you eat and to everything you drink. Not only does this enhance the nutritional value of the food, but it can also help to balance the ill effects of additives and chemicals and bring the food into harmony with your body. I personally like to use Reiki as a type of blessing, and it feels good to exchange some energy with our food, because everything we eat was a living thing, not just meat and fish. The vegetables, fruits, nuts and seeds were also living, if not in the same way, but they, too, have given up life to provide us with energy so that we may continue to live. It is therefore in line with the Reiki principles to be grateful for what we eat. You don't have to hold your hands over your food in an overt act—you can be discreet and hold your hands at the sides of your plate, or around the cup or glass just for a brief time—a few seconds is all that is needed—and you might like to say a little prayer of thanks either silently or out loud. The one I use is:

> I give Reiki to this food and drink in grateful thanks to the earth, the plants, the creatures and the people who have helped to bring me this nourishment. I also give Reiki to this food and drink to enhance its nutritional quality, and to bring it into harmony with my body so that it helps my body to be vibrantly well.

Healing the Planet

The earth really needs as much healing as we can give her, and with Reiki you have a wonderful tool to use for planetary healing. There are many methods for earth healing, and I give some suggestions below. Although all of them can be enhanced by using Reiki, you could also try some of these even if you don't do Reiki—simply use your thought energy, and imagine white light and healing going to the earth instead.

1. Go to a place of power, such as an ancient stone circle, and either sit in the middle, or place your hands on one of the stones, and allow Reiki to flow into the stone, around the circle and into the earth itself, *intending* that the Reiki flows for the greatest and highest good of the planet. You can also direct the Reiki to flow out of your feet, and you will often find that your feet get really hot when you do this.

2. Sit or stand either outdoors or indoors with your palms facing downward, and direct Reiki into the earth, *intending* that it be used by the planet for its greatest and highest good.

3. Imagine that you are holding a small version of the world between your hands, and send it Reiki.

4. Hold something in your hands to represent the earth, such as a stone, and fill it with Reiki, intending that the Reiki should fill the planet.

Using Reiki on World Situations and Disasters

Unfortunately, there are many negative situations in the world today, and to send Reiki to global situations, such as famines, ecological disasters or war zones, write down the situation and hold the piece of paper in your hands, *intending* that Reiki should go to that situation for the highest possible good—with Reiki 2 you can also draw the distant symbol over it to connect to that area, then the harmony symbol and the power symbol to bring harmony and healing to the situation for the greatest and highest good of all. In this way the Reiki is not being constrained to only go to one aspect of the situation, such as the people affected by the famine, but to the whole, so that it can also permeate the aid agencies, the governments, any warring factions, and so on. It really is gratifying to feel that you can do something to help, because so often we are too far removed from such situations to either fully understand them or offer practical assistance. Many thousands of people send Reiki to world situations every day, and if you have access to the Internet you may find websites or receive e-mails telling you about the latest healing "target" with which you can join in, if you wish.

Using Reiki with Plants and Seeds

Seeds and plants respond extremely well to being treated with Reiki, and I have tested this out many times. I have kept houseplants alive for months without water, just by giving them Reiki each day—and I don't just mean cacti or succulents, which like dry conditions. It has worked with "difficult" plants like poinsettias and maidenhair ferns. I have also tried planting seeds in identical compost and containers and given Reiki to only half the seeds. In each case those given Reiki grew much faster and more strongly than those that were not treated, and those planted in the Reiki half also had a 100 percent germination rate.

To give Reiki to seeds, simply hold the packet between your hands and *intend* that Reiki should flow to the seeds, or alternatively plant them and then hold your hands over the seed trays. For houseplants the easiest way is to hold your hands on each side of the pot for about a minute, or alternatively you can hold your hands about 15 centimeters (6 inches) away from the plant. In each case, if you have Reiki 2 you can use the power symbol, drawn either over the plant or seeds, or on the palms of your hands before giving the Reiki. If you have a lot of plants, a quick and easy idea is to Reiki the water you use when giving them their regular watering. This is even possible when watering a garden using a hose, as you can *intend* that as the water passes through the section of the hose you are holding, it will receive Reiki.

If you grow seedlings on your windowsill or in a greenhouse, or buy plants from garden centers, or wish to transplant something from one area of your garden to another, then as well as giving them a good soaking beforehand, Reiki them during the planting stage (using the harmony symbol as well as the power symbol if you have Reiki 2) and daily for at least a week afterward.

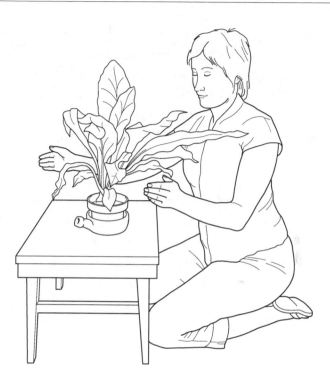

Also use Reiki on the water when you water the plants, and as often as possible afterward.

I am particularly fond of trees, and I would urge you to give Reiki to as many trees as you can at any time of the year, but particularly in the autumn and winter when their natural energy levels are low. They have an auric field that is quite similar to a human aura, and they respond really well to Reiki, sometimes coming into a second flowering, as if in gratitude. Try it!

Reiki and Inanimate Objects

It may stretch your credulity, but Reiki can work very well on inanimate objects like cars, computers and washing machines, and this isn't really as strange as it may sound. As mentioned in Chapter 4, everything in the universe is energy, and all "man-made" objects started out as natural materials. Those natural materials may have changed state, but they are still energy, and once energy has been created, it cannot be destroyed; it can only be transformed into some other state—think of water, which can be transformed into ice, steam or condensation, etc.

Again, this is something I have tried out on many occasions, and I have succeeded in getting dishwashers, vacuum cleaners, clocks and cars to work after they had broken down, and, even more useful at the time, getting my computer to work again after the system totally crashed and I really didn't have the time to reconfigure it before completing the document on which I was working. I even know of one case where a cell phone began to charge when Reiki was being used nearby! I'm not suggesting that Reiki should be used in place of regular maintenance—your car will still need service—and unfortunately it doesn't replace the need for diesel or gas either, but it is useful when things go wrong.

Using Reiki with Crystals

Before you use any kind of crystal, you should ensure that it has been cleansed. You may have heard of various methods of cleansing, but some can be detrimental to the crystals—for example, you should not place crystals in salt or in salt water, as this can erode some of the more delicate varieties. Also, it is not advisable to place uncleansed crystals in sunlight or moonlight, as this does not cleanse them, but empowers them, so if they are full of negative energy you are actually increasing the power

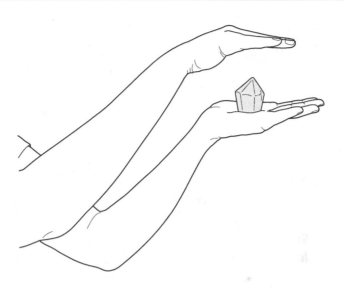

of that negativity. Running clean, cold water over crystals is quite good, especially in untreated water such as a stream or river, or even bottled mineral water. However, the best way to cleanse crystals is to use energy—you can use Reiki on a crystal simply by holding it in your hands and *intending* that the Reiki should cleanse it.

It is also possible to program crystals with Reiki so that they carry the healing energy, and I have found that clear quartz, rose quartz and amethyst are the best for this purpose. However, although it might feel strange at first, you should really ask permission from the crystal before programming it for healing. Just hold the cleansed crystal in your hands and mentally ask it if it is happy to be used for healing—if the answer is "no" you will usually either get a slightly uncomfortable tingle in your hands, or a slightly sick feeling in your solar plexus. If this happens, replace the crystal and use another one, following the same pattern of cleansing and asking permission, and if the answer is "yes" you will usually feel warmth in your hands or a good feeling in your solar plexus. (Other sensations do occur, such as coolness, buzzing, etc., but use your intuition to decide what feels right to you.) Then allow Reiki to flow into the crystal, and "program" it by *intending* that it should hold the healing energy and release it when required.

You can then carry the crystal around with you to aid your own healing, or give it to someone else who needs healing energy. You can also write down any problem you are experiencing on a piece of paper and place it under the crystal, *intending* that the Reiki flow constantly into the problem to create healing for the highest possible good. It is best to cleanse the crystal and reprogram it once a week to maintain the strength of the energy. If you have Reiki 2, you can draw the power symbol over the crystal—and if it has a number of facets, draw the power symbol over each facet, *intending* either that Reiki cleanse the crystal, or program it with healing, whichever is appropriate at that time.

Try holding your hand over a quartz crystal before programming it with Reiki, and then again afterward. You will be amazed at the power coming from the crystal after it has been filled with Reiki, which will usually make your hand tingle, particularly in the center of the palm.

The ideas listed in this chapter are just some of the ways in which Reiki can be used creatively, but there are many others, and I'm sure that none of us has yet discovered the full potential of Reiki. However, if more and more people start to use it, together we could heal the world. Now there's a thought!

chapter fourteen

REIKI WITH ANIMALS

Many people are very fond of animals, so if you are attuned to Reiki it can be an especially delightful and satisfying thing to extend your gift of healing energy to your pets. I even know some people who have chosen to specialize in treating animals in preference to treating people, and they deal with all types, from farm animals to wild creatures, and even fish, reptiles and insects. However, I would point out that in the UK, and possibly elsewhere, there are legal implications that apply to *any-one* treating animals. I provide details of these, given to me by the Royal College of Veterinary Surgeons in London, in the section on treating animals professionally (see page 242).

I have had some interesting experiences when using Reiki on animals, and hopefully in this chapter I can give you some ideas for the best and easiest ways to channel Reiki for the benefit of animals and other creatures. Of course Reiki is a wonderful healing tool for every living thing, and most types of animals respond to it very well in such an unquestioning and trustful way that it can be quite a humbling experience. It does seem that animals are very much more in tune with their own health and energy needs than humans, and they are also much more intuitive and can detect healing energies more easily than we can. Because of this they are often drawn to people whose energies they know will help them, so as a Reiki channel you may well find that you could become like the "pied piper" in the well-known fairy tale—although hopefully you won't attract just rats!

THE BASICS OF TREATING ANIMALS

First of all, let's look at the basic methods for using Reiki with animals. The way you treat a particular animal will obviously depend upon its size and temperament, and while with some you can follow a similar format of hand positions to those you would use on humans, with others you may need to use different methods depending upon specific circumstances. However, the six main approaches are as follows:

1. Placing the hands directly on the animal, whenever it is safe and practical to do so.
2. Placing the hands on the cage or tank in which the animal is housed, where the animal is too small or too dangerous to touch, or where direct touch would disadvantage the creature (e.g., a fish).
3. Holding a small animal in your hands, if this is safe to do, and won't frighten the creature too much.
4. Sending Reiki through the aura to an animal, either holding your hands directly above the animal, or from several yards away.
5. Using the Reiki symbols to direct Reiki to an animal,

which can be even more effective than the previous method.

6. Sending a full distant treatment to an animal, either as a one-off experience, or as a regular thing in the case of severe illness.

Most of the above methods will be familiar to you, but perhaps I had better explain about sending Reiki through your aura to an animal. As explained in Chapter 4, the energy field around your body can extend as much as 20 meters (66 feet) or more in front of you, and the same distance behind you, although 3–4.5 meters (10–15 feet) is probably more usual. This means that if you are standing up to 10 feet away from an animal, it is probably encompassed in your aura, so all you need to do is think and *intend* that Reiki is filling your aura, and it will do so, and the animal will then be surrounded by Reiki. You can then *intend* that the Reiki flows into the animal for its greatest and highest good, and if the animal is happy to receive it, that is what will happen.

Even if an animal is much further away, you can still connect to it in this way because it is possible to consciously push your aura out as far as you need it to go—even 500 meters (1,640 feet) or more—by visualizing the edge of your aura expanding until it is large enough for the animal to be inside it. Then let your aura fill with Reiki, as before, and allow the Reiki to flow into the animal's aura and from there into its body, if the animal is willing to receive it. (It is unlikely that the Reiki will be rejected, but there will be no harm done either way, because the Reiki will just work with your own aura if this happens, which is fine.) This method is an alternative to using the Reiki symbols to send Reiki, so it is a good way for people to work if they haven't done Reiki 2.

DEALING WITH PETS

The animals most people are keen to treat with Reiki are their pets, and the method you use will depend not only on the size of the animal, but also on the type of relationship you have with it. Dogs and cats are probably the most popular pets, and the ones people feel closest to, and generally they are the easiest to treat with Reiki. Any hand positions you choose will obviously depend upon where you can reach, and where the animal will allow you to touch, as well as where it is safe to touch—even pets can be bad-tempered sometimes, especially if they are in pain. Also remember that while some animals will happily sit or stand for a long time to receive Reiki, and keep coming back for more, others will quickly move away, or they may react quite differently if you attempt to touch any sensitive parts of their bodies. Even pets that would usually sit happily to be stroked or petted may walk off if you try to give them Reiki, and if that happens, allow them to go. I have seen enthusiastic Reiki students covered in scratches from their normally affectionate cat after frenzied and determined attempts to practice Reiki on their pet, when the animal clearly didn't want any.

Depending upon the size of the animal, you might try one or two hand positions on the head, and two or three on either side of the body. Some animals seem to dislike Reiki being given directly onto their spine, although cats can be an exception to this.

Normally if there is a specific injury, it is sensible to concentrate treatment on that area, but of course you need to take care not to touch directly any part that might cause the animal pain. There is no problem with this, because we know that Reiki will flow around the whole body, so wherever you place your hands the animal will draw sufficient Reiki into itself for its needs—and of course Reiki can enter the auric field and filter into the physical body from there, so you can hold your hands 5–8 centimeters (2–3 inches) or more above or near to the injury site, and the Reiki will flow in quite easily.

The amount of time required for treatment will vary greatly, and will depend upon the size of the animal as well as on the severity of any illness or injury. If you are treating a very small pet like a rabbit, guinea pig, hamster

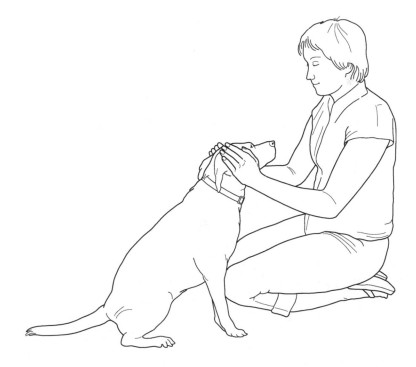

or gerbil, and if it is friendly enough, you might be able to hold it in your hands to give it Reiki, and because of its size it would probably need only 5–15 minutes. However, if the animal is in any way aggressive, it would be just as effective to hold your hands on or near its hutch or cage and just let the Reiki flow through your aura into the animal's aura, from where it would also flow into the animal's body.

If you have a pet bird, reptile or insect, they may be well used to you handling them, in which case you can just hold them between your hands and let the Reiki flow. However, if they are likely to peck, bite, scratch or sting you, it may be more circumspect to treat them in the cage, tank or hut where they live, or to put them in something like a shoe box (with air holes in it). Simply place your hands on or near the receptacle and *intend* that the Reiki should flow to the creature, and take your hands away when it feels appropriate to do so. Any small creatures will usually need treating for only a few minutes. Of course, if your pet needs more than one treatment, you can give it as much Reiki as you like—it isn't possible to overdose on Reiki. Pet fish must obviously be treated in their normal environment—i.e., with your hands placed on or near their bowl or tank, ensuring that the water is at the appropriate temperature and salinity.

USING REIKI ON YOUR ANIMAL'S FOOD AND MEDICATION

Another good way to help your pets, or any other animals you are caring for, is to use Reiki on their food and water to enhance its nutritional qualities and to offset any adverse effects of any chemicals or preservatives. This is simple to do. Hold the food or water bowl with one hand under it and one hand over it, and *intend* that Reiki should flow into it. You can also do this with a box, packet or can of food in your hands, *intending* that Reiki should flow into it—a minute is usually enough, and 30 seconds will probably do. Any homeopathic remedies or medication dispensed by a veterinary surgeon can also be given Reiki in the same way.

USING REIKI ON HORSES AND FARM ANIMALS

Many people have as close a relationship with their horses as others do with their dogs or cats, so treating them is generally fairly easy as they are used to human contact. It is possible to treat a horse with Reiki while sitting astride it, so you can place your hands on either side of the head, neck and flanks, but otherwise it is probably easiest to stand beside the horse and move down one side, placing your hands wherever you feel is appropriate, and then do roughly the same positions on the other side. Horses' legs and feet are often prone to injury, so these can be treated using both hands in much the same way as you would a human leg—but humans don't tend to kick as hard as horses, so do be particularly wary when doing this.

Of course, you don't have to own or work with horses to feel sympathy if you see a dejected or ill-looking horse in a field—and I do think that Reiki makes us more able

241

to intuit when something is wrong with an animal. Sadly, many horses are ill-treated, either deliberately or because their owners are ignorant about the correct way to look after them, so I have sometimes felt it necessary to stop at the roadside, beside a hedge or fence, and let my aura expand until it encompasses a horse which is obviously in distress. Often after ten minutes or so the horse will begin to raise its head, and will slowly amble over to me, putting its head over the fence so that I can place my hands on it. The gentleness and trust it shows when doing this is quite awesome to me, because under normal circumstances I am a bit nervous around horses. Alternatively, if I don't have much time to stop, I have used the distant symbol to connect with the horse and sent Reiki to it using the power symbol, *intending* that it receive as much Reiki as it needs—and of course you can do this with several horses at the same time, if you have done Reiki 2.

It is often easiest to treat farm animals such as cattle, sheep, pigs, hens or geese through the aura from the edge of the field or beside the pen, sty or other enclosure, either by expanding your aura, or by using the distant symbol to connect to them and the power symbol to enable the Reiki to flow.

TREATING ANIMALS PROFESSIONALLY

If you feel drawn to working professionally with animals, you must be aware of and abide by any laws relating to their treatment. According to the Royal College of Veterinary Surgeons, in the UK the Veterinary Surgeons

Act of 1966 states that anyone treating animals must be a qualified veterinary surgeon, and that no one other than a qualified vet can diagnose problems, carry out tests for diagnostic purposes, advise or carry out medical or surgical treatment or prescribe medication. Indeed, Section 19 makes it an offense for anyone other than a veterinary surgeon (or a veterinary student) to practice veterinary surgery. I've summarized what can be done legally in the chart below:

A: Provisions in Schedule 3 to the Veterinary Surgeons Act 1966

Subject	What may be done	By whom	Subject to what conditions
Treatment by owners (Sch. 3, para. 1)	Minor medical treatment	Owner, member of household, employee	
Farm animals (Sch. 3, para. 2, & SI 1991/1412)	Medical treatment or minor surgery not involving entry into body cavity	Owner, veterinary nurse, or person engaged or employed in caring for animal used in agriculture	Not done for reward
Emergencies (Sch. 3, para. 3)	First aid	Anyone	In emergency, to save life or relieve pain or suffering

So basically, unless you are already qualified as a veterinary surgeon or a veterinary nurse, or are an agricultural worker dealing with farm animals, or are treating your own pets, you are probably breaking the law if you treat an animal with Reiki, even if you have been on a specific course purporting you to be qualified to treat animals with Reiki.

However, it does appear to be legal for anyone to treat their own animals, or to treat an animal in an emergency, and clearly it would be difficult to legislate against anyone giving distant Reiki to an animal, but if you do decide to treat any animals other than your own with Reiki it is essential that you advise the animal's owner(s) to register the animal with a qualified veterinary surgeon, and you must advise them to take their animal to that vet for diagnosis and treatment. Regulations in other countries may be different, but I would advise you to check them before carrying out any work with animals.

TREATING WILD ANIMALS

Wild animals, including birds, frequently get injured on our roads or in other areas close to human habitation, so you might come across some and wish to help. Birds and other small animals are probably best placed in a cardboard box with air holes before being treated, as contact with humans can be very frightening, and the shock can even cause some to die—and if the injury is serious, it is obviously best to transport the animal as quickly as you can to a vet or animal clinic. If you should ever need to give Reiki to an animal that might prove dangerous (e.g., in a zoo), or is too nervous to let you get near it, then it is perfectly acceptable to stand a safe distance away and send the Reiki through your own aura into the auric field of the animal, or to use the distant symbol to connect with it and then the power symbol to bring the Reiki powerfully to it. By using the Second Degree Reiki symbols you can probably see the possibilities already—it means that no injured, sick, suffering, agitated or dangerous creature will be unable to receive help. You can connect with an individual animal, or in the case of herd or pack animals whose consciousness is linked, you can connect with the whole group to send Reiki, for their greatest and highest good.

COMMUNICATING WITH ANIMALS

As mentioned, I do think Reiki helps us to sense more easily when animals are ill or distressed, but I think it also helps us to develop a greater awareness of their needs—to be able to communicate with them. I first became interested in communicating with animals when my daughter read a book by Sonya Fitzpatrick (*What the Animals Tell Me: Developing Your Innate Telepathic Skills to Understand and Communicate with Your Pets*) and passed it on to me. I've used the techniques quite often, and they really do work. Basically, Sonya Fitzpatrick points out that animals are telepathic, and they pick up the images in our thoughts, rather than the words we use—which is why our pets know when we're about to arrive home, or go on vacation, or take them to the vet, because we visualize what we think about. It is also one of the ways in which they pick up on our moods, so a dog or cat will often be especially affectionate if we are upset, for instance.

You can prepare your pet in advance of your absence by sitting with them and visualizing yourself going away, perhaps by car, and then visualizing the sun going down, and then rising again for the number of days you are going away, until you finally "see" yourself coming home and greeting your pet. I've used this method successfully many times, and proved its effectiveness when I was once away for longer than expected, and my cat, which had until then been perfectly content, became agitated and stopped eating for the last few days of my absence.

CALMING ANIMALS

Another excellent use of Reiki is for helping to calm animals when they are angry, anxious or distressed, and I have found this useful in a number of situations, including an occasion when I found myself in a field with a rather angry-looking bull. Sending Reiki to it using the distant symbol, the harmony symbol and the power symbol had the desired effect—it looked a bit puzzled, then lay down and started chewing the cud—giving me the time to make a reasonably rapid escape. This technique can also work on other animals, such as dogs, but I would always advise caution—it's much better to move away if possible, to avoid confrontation. However, using the harmony symbol with any animal can reduce its anxiety, so if your pet has to travel, or if you are taking it to the vet or moving home with it, then a short Reiki treatment beforehand, using the harmony symbol as well as the power symbol, can help to prepare it. Visualizing it traveling happily and arriving safely, perhaps finishing with an image of a bowl of its favorite food, will be helpful, too, as it will telepathically pick up on those images.

HEALING PROJECTS WITH ANIMALS

Hopefully this chapter has given you some ideas on how you can use Reiki with your pets and other animals, but you don't have to limit yourself to working with animals that are known to you. You could create a healing project for yourself, perhaps sending Reiki regularly for a month to all the animals in your nearest zoo, for their greatest and highest good. The next month you could send Reiki to the whales and dolphins in the coastal waters or deep-sea areas near to the country in which you live, or elsewhere in the world. After that you could send Reiki out generally to be received by any animals that are being mistreated, and so on. Whatever you decide to do, using Reiki with animals is a very worthwhile and beautiful way of working with this wonderful healing energy we are lucky enough to be able to channel.

PROGRESSING IN REIKI

In this part of the book we have discussed many different ways of using Reiki, but some people are interested in taking their Reiki further by becoming either Reiki practitioners, or Reiki Masters/teachers, and that is what I cover in Part 5.

part five

PROGRESSING IN REIKI

chapter fifteen

BECOMING A REIKI PRACTITIONER

Some months or even years after you start treating family and friends with Reiki, you might begin to think of becoming a professional Reiki practitioner, using your healing skills in either a voluntary or a paid capacity on a more formal basis. This can be a very rewarding and interesting step to take, but as mentioned in Chapter 9, the training required in the future, at least in the UK, will be more extensive than it has been previously. While this might make it a longer process and harder work for the potential practitioner in order to comply with registration requirements, it will lead to much better practice and a safer and even more effective experience for the clients. It will also mean that, after their training and assessment, those working in the UK will have the benefit of being included on a national register of Reiki practitioners, so that clients will be able to find them more easily than they can now. However, before you make the decision to progress to professional practice, it might be useful to look at what is involved.

YOUR PERSONAL "SWOT" ANALYSIS

If you've never done any business or management training, you're probably thinking "What is a SWOT?" but it
isn't as odd as it sounds. The letters stand for Strengths,
Weaknesses, Opportunities and Threats, and it is a way of
assessing where you are, right now, and what else you
need in order to be successful. The simplest way is to take
a sheet of paper and divide it evenly into four squares,
writing one of the words at the top of each square, and
then jot down all your ideas in each section.

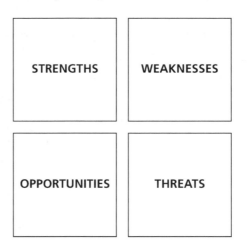

- **Strengths** These could be being good with people,
  well organized and tidy, paying attention to detail,
  being committed to Reiki, having a spare room that
  could be turned into a therapy room, or already having qualifications in other therapies and thus being
  able offer a range of treatments, etc.
- **Weaknesses** These could include not being good
  with money, not knowing how to keep accounts,
  being rather shy, not yet having a proper massage

table, having young children who will need baby-sitters when you're practicing, being difficult to get to on public transport, etc.

◆ **Opportunities** These could include the possibility that there is no one in your area currently offering Reiki, that your local doctor has a policy of being "friendly" toward complementary therapies, so they may be willing to refer people to you, that a brand-new holistic center is opening up nearby, that there are various local groups to which you could give short talks and demonstrations about Reiki to get people interested—or that you have just won the lottery, so you can have your own, purpose-built clinic!

◆ **Threats** These could be that there are already four Reiki practitioners in your area, that there is a "free" healing group nearby two evenings a week, or that the local holis-tic center has put up posters advertising Reiki courses.

The idea is to get a realistic overview of your potential, so that if there are areas you need to improve, you can do something about it, and if there are aspects you could make even better use of, you can make sure you exploit those opportunities. Get some ideas and support from family and friends, too, as they might be affected by you setting out on a new career.

THE RESPONSIBILITY OF PRACTITIONER STATUS

When you first start practicing on friends and family, even though you may be very professional about it, it isn't the same as working as a practitioner, taking clients who will probably initially be strangers to you. People who have not met you before will expect certain standards from you, and will regard you with respect as a "health professional." They may well expect you to have considerable medical or therapeutic knowledge and experience, and may judge you against other therapists they have known. All of this will seem very different from giving your mom, brother or best friend a treatment.

What is important, however, is that you develop—and stick to—your own high standards of behavior and professional practice, ensuring that you do everything you can to treat people politely, sensitively, and with great care and attention. You should also ensure that each client has as comfortable—and comforting—an experience as possible, so you will need to pay attention to the environment you are providing, as well as to the way in which you talk to the client before and after the treatment, and the way you carry out the treatment itself. In fact, all of these points are covered in the National Occupation Standards (NOS) for Reiki (see also page 265), so they provide plenty of guidance on what standards you need to be aiming for.

GAINING PRACTICE AND EXPERIENCE

It is obviously sensible to get plenty of practice and experience before you start practicing professionally, partly because it will help to give you confidence, since any potential clients will expect you to know what you're doing, and if you feel unsure, so will they. Another reason is because the more you practice, the better able you will be to understand and detect subtle energies, and to give each individual client what they need. It isn't just about placing your hands in 12 different places for five minutes each. As your experience grows you will sense that some areas need more time, some need less; also, some clients need more time to talk before and after treatment, while others prefer as little communication as possible.

The more you practice and self-treat, the better a channel you will be for Reiki, and the more Reiki your future clients will be able to receive. Also, if you wish to become a UK-registered Reiki practitioner, you will need to have completed plenty of treatments before registration can be achieved. It is therefore important that you keep records of all the treatments you do, preferably from the very beginning (i.e., Reiki 1) so that they can be counted toward your total experience.

WHAT DOES IT TAKE TO BE A GOOD PRACTITIONER?

If you go to a therapist of any kind, what sort of experience do you hope you will have, and how do you want to be treated? Whatever your answer is, that is what it takes to be a good practitioner. Unfortunately, a proficient practitioner needs to be all things to all people, which is a pretty tall order. It means you need to be a good listener, to have an understanding and caring nature, to be empathetic and sympathetic with people and treat them with respect, but also to be knowledgeable, confident and firm enough to command their respect. And of course, you also need to be thoroughly experienced and good at what you do.

So being experienced in the practice of Reiki isn't all it takes. You also need to be competent in a wide range of other abilities, especially those that help you to deal with people, for instance coping with clients in the midst of an emotional release, which can be one of the effects of a Reiki treatment. You may therefore wish to acquire some knowledge, experience and qualifications in related skills, such as counseling or NLP to help with this side of your practice (see also page 157).

Good communication skills enable a practitioner to be supportive and positive, so that they can encourage a healthy self-belief and a sense of self-empowerment in their clients. When a client can begin to take part in their own healing, taking constructive action toward good health practices, they will usually respond better to treatments, and make even greater progress in their overall health.

Another aspect of being a good practitioner is your organizational skills. You could be a wonderfully empathetic therapist who channels Reiki beautifully, but if you don't keep adequate records, and provide a clean and tidy environment, and if you're never ready when a client arrives, or, worse, you aren't even there because you'd forgotten to write the appointment on your calendar, then you won't be seen as a good practitioner.

CODES OF ETHICS AND CONDUCT

When you are working as a Reiki practitioner the most important ethical considerations are integrity, respect and confidentiality. Your behavior must be seen to demonstrate all of these, in order for your clients to be able to develop respect for you and trust in you. Needless to say, practitioners must never give the impression that they have medical qualifications if they do not.

To act with integrity, you must make clear to your clients—before starting a treatment—what is involved in a Reiki treatment, how long it will last and how much it will cost, and you should explain to them what type of client records you keep. You may not be able to discuss how many consultations you think may be necessary, at least until after the first treatment, but you should always leave the option open for your clients not to take your advice—ultimately it is up to them how many times they come for treatments. However, it is absolutely vital that you do *not* offer any diagnoses, and do *not* claim or promise a cure. The person's Soul/Higher Self decides the amount of healing required at an unconscious level, and the Reiki is directed by a Higher Consciousness to those areas with the greatest need. Promising miracle cures is unethical, illegal and dangerous, because you could be falsely raising hopes. Yes, miracles do happen, but no one knows when—or why.

If at any time you feel that a client should consult a doctor, you can suggest this, but do so in as calm and respectful a manner as possible. For example, perhaps you felt a lump or an unexpected mass when you placed your hands on some part of the client's body, or you had a particularly strong flow of Reiki for a long time in one place. Obviously, it would be appropriate to treat that area with plenty of Reiki, but afterward it would also be appropriate to gently ask the client if they had detected any problems in that area, and to calmly suggest that they see a doctor to reassure themselves, as it is always sensible to have such things checked out. Don't, under any circumstances, be drawn into saying what you think it might be. The best answer is always, "I'm sorry, I'm not a doctor, so I have no idea. The best thing to do is to get it checked"—unless, of course, you happen to be a doctor of medicine. However, although it is not illegal for someone to refuse to seek medical advice, you must write in the client's notes that you have advised them to do so.

When using Reiki on clients who are receiving conventional medical treatment, you should *never* advise them to stop taking any medicines, reduce their medication or stop seeing their doctor or other health professional. However, if a client is on medication to restore balance in the body, for conditions such as diabetes or high blood pressure, you should advise them to keep a close eye on their self-monitoring results and to check these regularly with their doctor in case they need their medication dosage changed. This is because Reiki can often help the body to reach a more appropriate balance, so it can (but does not always) result in some positive changes.

(Some people within the Reiki community believe that there might be contraindications if Reiki is used under certain circumstances, for instance when a client has a pacemaker, or if they are also receiving radiation treatment or chemotherapy, but as Reiki always works for the greatest and highest good, I personally don't believe it can do any harm—but you must do what you feel is right.)

Another thing to remember is that clients may be

nervous when coming for a treatment, so it is important to treat them with gentleness and respect, and to invite them to ask questions and discuss anything about the treatment that may be worrying them. You will then be able to reassure them so that they can relax and enjoy the treatment.

RECORD KEEPING

You should keep records of every client you treat, for every visit. These records should be simple, straightforward and free from any personal views or judgments, and they should be stored in accordance with the current laws on data protection in whichever country you work. The basic information required is:

1. Personal information: name, address, telephone number, date of birth and details of someone to contact in an emergency.
2. Reason for receiving Reiki: Why is the person seeking Reiki? It should be noted that while a person may request help for a particular condition, Reiki may or may not address this problem.
3. Comfort needs: any specific physical requirements that may affect the comfort of the client.
4. Interaction with allopathic or complementary treatments: Is the client taking regular medication or having treatments with another practitioner? If so, it is good practice to advise them to inform their doctor/ practitioner that they are receiving Reiki as well. A note of such advice should be made.

5. Possible reactions: Are there other conditions practitioners should be aware of so that they can advise the client appropriately and be well prepared to meet the individual's needs?
6. Other relevant information: anything else they feel it is important to tell you.

It is your duty to keep all information relating to each client entirely confidential (even from members of their own family) if you do not have the client's consent to divulge it, unless you are legally obliged to do so by a court of law. This not only refers to any medical information the client might share with you, but also to any records you hold which refer to them and details of their appointments with you. A possible exception to this is if you believe there is a threat of suicide, which you are legally bound to report to an appropriate health professional such as a doctor or psychiatrist.

You also need to ensure that you comply with the current Data Protection Act and any other current relevant legislation with regard to the storage of data, and must keep all your client records under lock and key. You should even make arrangements in your will for what should happen to those records if you die. If you are practicing outside the UK, check what regulations apply in your country.

PREMISES AND EQUIPMENT

You will need somewhere to practice, and there are a number of options. You could work from home if you have a suitable room that can be totally private from the rest of the household (but do check with your landlord/ mortgage holder/local council first), or you could hire a room in a holistic therapy center, or even a hair-dresser's or beautician's. Alternatively, you could operate as a mobile therapist, working in your clients' homes. This is reasonably easy because you need very little equipment in order to practice Reiki, other than a stationary or portable massage table. These are available in various heights, widths and weights, and at a range of prices, so you should be able to find one that is suitable for you.

LEGAL RESPONSIBILITIES

Insurance

You will need to be adequately insured to practice, so you must have public liability insurance, public indemnity and malpractice insurance and, if you employ anyone else, employee liability insurance as well. It is good practice to have these certificates available, or even discreetly displayed somewhere in your therapy room. Insurance can usually be obtained at a reasonable cost through an umbrella organization such as the UK Reiki Federation or the Reiki Association (see page 281), and there are relevant organizations in other countries that provide a similar service to their members.

Accounts, Insurance and Tax

It is essential to keep accounts, although these do not need to be complicated. A simple two-column system will suffice, as shown below, providing that you keep all your receipts and other paperwork regarding your business, such as bank statements, check stubs, credit and debit card slips and statements, invoices, gift certificates, and so on. Good record keeping pays dividends, because you will have to calculate how much tax you must pay, and if you haven't recorded all your necessary expenditures you will end up paying too much tax.

Income			Expenditure		
Date	Description	Amount	Date	Description	Amount

Even if you decide to use an accountant to prepare your records and tax returns, you will still need all of the above, so it is best to get into good habits right from the start.

Medical Restrictions and Notifiable Diseases

There are a surprising number of rules and regulations regarding what you can and cannot do as a health practitioner, and it is essential that you get up-to-date information about any legal requirements or regulations about medical restrictions and notifiable diseases for any country in which you wish to practice—ignorance of the law is no defense. Your professional association should be able to help you with this, and government websites also often

have useful information—you don't want to treat someone with Reiki and find that by doing so you could
be going against the law. (See also my book *The Reiki
Manual*.)

MARKETING

To get your business off to a good start—and to keep it
going—you will need to do at least a small amount of
marketing, to make sure that people know where you
are and what you do. There are a number of ways of
bringing your services to the attention of other people,
although by far the most effective is word of mouth. If
you always ensure that you give your clients a good
experience, they will often come back for more treatments themselves, and will usually recommend you to
their friends and relatives, too, and this will help to
increase your client base.

Advertising in local newspapers is rarely effective and
quite costly, so I would recommend that you limit any
advertising to specific publications dedicated to alternative therapies, although even these aren't often successful
in bringing you clients unless they are locally based.

You are unlikely to need expensively produced bro-
chures, or even business cards, but fairly simple leaflets and
flyers giving information about you, about Reiki, and
about the location, duration and cost of your treatments
are a good idea. These could be left at libraries, health-
food shops, holistic therapy centers, and so on, and do
put a poster in your local newsdealer's window, as this
can be very effective.

Leaflets, posters and flyers can be produced at home if you have a computer and a good printer, especially if you have a desktop publishing package, although do try to make it look as professional as possible. Also, get someone else to proofread it, as it can be difficult to spot your own mistakes—poor spelling and grammar can put people off, and anyway, they make you look at the very least careless, and at worst unprofessional.

Also remember that Reiki is not about competition—you need to trust in your potential for success, knowing that you will attract the right clients for you. The energy you put out will draw to you the people for whom you are exactly the right practitioner, so even if there is another Reiki practitioner nearby, they will attract whoever is right for them, too. Just use Reiki on the situation, and visualize nice, friendly people coming to you, and that's what you will get.

Of course, you don't have to start practicing Reiki full-time—you can always start in a very simple way, perhaps working one or two evenings a week, and gradually build up your business as you build up your confidence. And remember, you can use Reiki on all aspects of setting up a business, from attracting the right number of clients, to attracting the appropriate funding, premises or equipment.

TAKING A PROFESSIONAL QUALIFICATION

I talked about this in Chapter 9, and have briefly mentioned it again in some of the above sections, but from now onward in the UK you will need further training and experience after your attunement to Reiki before you can become a registered practitioner. This also is true for people who are already working as Reiki practitioners, although they should be able to count much of their previous experience toward the full qualification, using Accreditation of Prior Learning (APL).

As I said in Chapter 9, some Reiki Masters may be able to deliver all of the training required by the National Occupational Standards for Reiki, but it is likely that many will choose to carry on teaching Reiki in the way they currently do, and hand over the rest of the qualification process to individuals with specific skills, to Reiki organizations who could organize suitable workshops, or to colleges that already offer generic skills courses in appropriate subject areas such as health and safety or first aid.

NATIONAL OCCUPATIONAL STANDARDS FOR REIKI

All of the points I have dealt with in this chapter—codes of ethics, legal responsibilities, record keeping, premises, equipment, showing empathy for clients, and so on, are dealt with under the National Occupation Standards for Reiki in even more depth, so if you do intend to practice professionally, you will need to find out the most up-to-date information about what will be required. Basically, it will be up to the individual preregistered practitioners to take responsibility for their own learning and development, but it is empowering for practitioners to be responsible for their own research into professional practice standards. Later in this chapter and under Resources (see page 281), I refer to a number of websites that contain current information, as clearly there may be a few modifications over the years.

There are currently 12 different areas of competence identified in the NOS. Seven of these are compulsory and five are optional, and in order to achieve registration as a Reiki practitioner, people will have to complete eight competencies in total—all seven mandatory competencies, and then one chosen from the five optional competencies. It would then be possible to choose to complete some of the other optional competencies later, as part of their continuing professional development, if they wish.

The National Occupational Standards

These were developed through a process of discussion and consultation between the RRWG (now the Reiki Council) and Skills for Health, the UK's health-sector Skills Council. They outline the minimum knowledge and understanding you need in order to fulfill your obligations as a professional Reiki practitioner. They currently cover three main areas of practice, two of which are common to all complementary therapies:

CNH1 – Explore and establish the client's needs for complementary and natural health care.

CNH2 – Develop and agree on plans for complementary and natural health care with clients.

CNH12 – Provide Reiki to clients.

However, the relevant knowledge, training and experience you need can be roughly divided into the following topic areas:

Knowledge of Reiki

What style of Reiki you practice, including its history and your lineage, what "healing" is, how to carry out self-treatments and treatments on others, and how to provide Reiki to clients. This includes preparation, initial discussions, after-treatment advice, and when it would be inappropriate to give Reiki.

Anatomy and Physiology

Basic knowledge of the skeletal structure, the functions and locations of major organs, and the nature of common illnesses, as well as the ability to identify "red flag" symptoms and notifiable diseases.

Communicating with Clients

Basic understanding of verbal, nonverbal and written communication, such as discussing a client's needs, questioning and listening skills, interpreting body language, plus writing information in client records.

Practice Management

Providing suitable premises and equipment, being aware of health and safety needs, appropriate pricing, marketing and publicity, making appointments and keeping records, and taking care of yourself.

Fulfilling the Criteria for Registration

Accreditation for registration will probably be achieved in a number of ways, but any individual would be required to meet the requirements of the National Occupational Standards. This could be gained by attending accredited courses, or by Accreditation of Prior Learning (APL), which would be evidence based and could include testimonials, case histories, course certificates, journals or other methods of demonstrating the level of competence acquired. These could be assessed, and either the individual could then be registered, or any points for further attention identified. The benefits of this system would safeguard against "conveyor-belt" teaching of Reiki, and it would mean the student taking responsibility for meeting registration requirements, but there would be some flexibility in approach and in the time each individual took to reach the required standards. They would be free to find their own path with one or more Reiki Masters, and some aspects, such as health and safety, business acumen, first aid, etc., could be learned from other appropriate sources, not necessarily a Reiki teacher.

It is possible that complete courses may be accredited, which would offer a relatively simple route to registration, but as Reiki is not a practice that can be taught over a prescribed period of time, these would need to be modular, offering the potential for periods of pause to enable self-reflection that would facilitate the emotional and spiritual development of the student. These courses could be provided by individual Reiki Masters, Reiki organizations or perhaps by Reiki Masters teaching in colleges.

Students would maintain ongoing professional relationships with their Reiki teachers throughout the training period, and should have the opportunity to access continued support after completion of practitioner training. They will be expected to comply with all aspects of the National Occupational Standards (Reiki NOS), have a knowledge and understanding of the Code of Ethics and

Practice for Reiki practitioners in the UK, and have at least six months' Reiki experience following attunement/initiation.

Training as a Reiki Practitioner in Other Countries

The above practices will apply only in the UK, so if you live and work in other countries I would advise you to look into the legal position there (see Resources, page 281). For example, in some states in the U.S.A. it is illegal to use hands-on healing (including Reiki) unless you are a qualified minister or priest, and the legal position of Reiki in some European countries is that you have to be medically qualified before practicing Reiki professionally. Some other countries, notably Australia, have investigated the possibility of creating a national qualification in Reiki, although there are no firm resolutions yet, but I think it is probable that eventually others will follow Britain's lead so that the practice of Reiki can become even more widely accepted.

COMBINING REIKI WITH OTHER COMPLEMENTARY THERAPIES

Reiki works well with virtually all complementary therapies, but particularly well with any "hands-on" therapy, such as aromatherapy, reflexology, shiatsu, chiropractic, osteopathy and any other disciplines involving massage or manipulation. If you practice any of the above therapies and you are attuned to Reiki, then the energy will often automatically flow from your hands during the complementary therapy session, if the client needs it.

Remember, it is the client's Higher Self that decides how much Reiki they need, and where the Reiki goes to, so at this level the practitioner only needs to be willing to let the energy flow.

For therapies that entail taking some form of preparation internally, such as homeopathy, Bach Flower Remedies and herbal medicine, the bottle or container can be held in the hands to allow Reiki to flow into the medication. When doing this, it is usual to have the *intention* that Reiki should flow into the remedy, and the easiest way is to say to yourself (silently or aloud), "Let Reiki flow into this remedy to enhance its effectiveness, for the highest possible good." Reiki is always given for the highest possible good, and this effectively releases the practitioner from any particular expectations of, or responsibility for, what the Reiki will do.

If you do decide to become a Reiki practitioner, I wish you lots of success, and hope you find it to be a very fulfilling occupation. However, you may at some time also consider taking further Reiki training (Reiki Third Degree/Reiki 3) to become a Reiki Master, and that is what I cover in the next chapter.

chapter sixteen

BECOMING A REIKI MASTER

Becoming a Reiki Master can be a truly wonderful and life-enhancing experience, but as I said in Chapter 7, it certainly isn't just about gaining an extra qualification. The title Reiki Master was adopted in the West as a rough translation of the Japanese word "Sensei," meaning respected teacher, and to become a respected teacher of Reiki really means making a lifelong commitment to self-discovery, spiritual development and self-mastery, because no one can ever truly "master" the divine energy that is Reiki. I believe that the decision to train as a Reiki Master should not be taken lightly, or without adequate thought and preparation, because the process of becoming a Reiki Master can be physically, mentally, emotionally and spiritually demanding, even when you are sure it is a vital step on your spiritual path to enlightenment.

If that sounds a bit scary, I apologize. Or then again, maybe I don't. Because what I'm trying to do is to get you to understand the significance of such a decision. My view is that deciding to become a Reiki Master should probably rank alongside deciding to become a parent in terms of how seriously you should think about it. Both are lifetime roles.

Okay, I know sometimes having a baby can happen without you planning it, but for the most part you just have to make the best of things and simply get on with being a mother or a father—and almost always you learn to love the child anyway. Well, similarly, sometimes people become Reiki Masters without giving it much thought. But eventually the enormity and responsibility of what they have taken on will become clear, and by then it can come as a pretty big shock. However, just like having an unplanned baby, most people come to love being a Reiki Master, because it is one of the most rewarding, fascinating and fulfilling life roles you can have.

CHOOSING YOUR TYPE OF TRAINING AND INITIATING MASTER

Reiki Master training in the West varies enormously, from a short course that could be anything from one day to a week or more—although the most usual is three days—to an individual apprenticeship, working alongside a qualified Master for about a year. The cost of training as a Master varies enormously, too, from less than £100 ($180) to £6,000 ($10,000). However, you can't necessarily assume that a Master charging a high price is a good teacher offering high-quality instruction, or that one charging a low price is an ineffective teacher offering poor instruction—there are as many variations in Reiki Masters as there are in any other profession. There are some excellent Reiki teachers who charge moderate prices, whereas there are others who have little experience and offer inadequate information and poor support, yet who charge high prices. It is very much up to you to decide which is which.

What you need to consider is what sort of training suits you best. For example, do you prefer to learn in a group, or on a one-on-one basis? Would you like to work through all the theory on your own before attending a course, or do you like a more intensive approach? Obviously, a longer training tends to be more thorough, although some Masters issue their students very comprehensive manuals, and some even have CDs and DVDs to augment the in-person teaching.

What I would hope is that you don't let the cost be the major factor in your decision. Just as I believe Reiki finds you when the time is right, so I believe that the money you need to attend the Master training of your choice will turn up just when you need it. It's all down to the universal law of abundance—or what is sometimes called "cosmic ordering"—so if you really need something, and it is for your highest and greatest good, you just need to ask, and you will receive it. So many students have told me amazing stories of how the money just turned up out of the blue, often from a totally unexpected source, and my own experience of such things also confirms it.

Obviously, the way in which Reiki Masters train other Masters will depend upon how they trained, with perhaps some individual differences based upon their experience since becoming qualified themselves. For example, some Masters insist that you should have at least three years' experience of Reiki, preferably as a professional practitioner, before they will accept you for Master training, while others have no minimum time requirements, and some even actively encourage every student to become a Reiki Master as soon as possible.

You can therefore choose to take the fast track, or the slow and easy route, taking as much time as you feel you need between initiations. Whichever you choose is always at the right speed at a Soul level—because at that level it isn't possible to make mistakes, since all experience is valid. However, I feel I need to point out that for some people, rushing through the levels can have some rather unpleasant consequences at the human level, because while your aura can expand and adjust fairly easily to the higher vibrational frequencies of the Reiki at each attunement level, your physical body, and your emotional and mental bodies, find it harder to adapt quickly to such huge changes in energy. This can therefore lead to a rapid (and potentially uncomfortable) cleansing period, not only of your physical body, but also of all areas of your life.

WHAT TO LOOK FOR IN THE TRAINING

There are obviously some basics that *must* be included in Reiki Master training, and other aspects that would be an advantage, but which are not essential. I have put together a short checklist which you might find useful when making your decision on where to go for training.

Essentials

- Receiving the Usui Reiki Master attunement.
- Learning the Usui Reiki Master symbol and its mantra, and how to use it (e.g., in treatments, distant healing and attunements).
- What to include when teaching Reiki at First Degree, Second Degree and Master levels.
- Learning (and practicing) the attunement processes for each level.
- The spiritual and business responsibilities of being a Reiki Master, and your ongoing responsibility for personal and spiritual development.

Useful Extras

- The traditional Japanese Reiju spiritual empowerment methods.
- The two additional symbols and mantras from William Lee Rand's Usui/Tibetan system, and methods for using them (e.g., balancing the chakras and clearing the aura).
- The Usui/Tibetan attunement processes for each level (these are different from the traditional Usui method).

Depending upon the amount of time available, there are other things that can be fun to learn, and that enhance the training experience, such as special meditations, energy cleansing with smudge sticks, empowering crystals, etc. Other opportunities may also be offered, such as observation and coteaching of Reiki 1 and Reiki 2 courses with your initiating Master. Also, you may find that some Masters divide the training into several parts, calling the first part Master Practitioner and the second part Master Teacher, so on the first course you are taught and attuned to the Usui Master symbol, and receive instruction in a few techniques, and on the second course you are trained in the attunement processes so that you can teach and attune others. (If your Reiki Master uses the Usui/Tibetan system, they would normally call the first part Advanced Reiki Training, or ART.)

Something to be aware of is that a significant proportion of Reiki Masters in the West don't actually use—or teach—the original Usui system for attunements, and some don't even teach the Usui Master symbol, or attune you to it. This is because so many Reiki Masters have been taught in the "modern" way, on short courses lasting between one and three days, using the Usui/Tibetan system originated by William Lee Rand. This does bring through a wonderful healing energy, but it is somewhat "fiercer" than the very gentle, flowing Usui Reiki energy, so you might like to ask any Master you intend working with which system they use, and perhaps experience an attunement from them (at Reiki 1 or 2) before making your decision to train further with them. And I would always advise you to ask your potential Reiki Master as many questions as you like—it is a very important step you are thinking of taking, so you need to be sure you've found the right person. Liking and respecting them is really essential, as hopefully it will be the start of a long-term supportive relationship.

AFTER A REIKI MASTER COURSE

The first and most important thing to remember is that receiving a Master attunement does not make you a

Reiki Master. It is just the beginning of a long journey *toward* the mastery of Reiki—a journey without end, because this amazing, divinely guided energy is beyond mastery by humans. But we can do our best to live up to it, to "walk our talk," to gradually "become" Reiki, so that it forms a vital and inexorable part of our lives.

At Master level, personal and spiritual development is no longer an option—it is a necessity. Reiki will lead you toward a more spiritual way of being, through experiences that will give you a greater level of wisdom and understanding about yourself and about other people. To become a Reiki Master is to become the *embodiment* of Reiki—the embodiment of love, light, healing, harmony and balance. That might seem pretty daunting, especially at first, but at a Soul level you always make the right decisions, so when you decide to become a Reiki Master it is always the right time.

It's a good idea to take the pressure off yourself, and not decide straightaway when you're going to begin attuning other people. Take some time to get used to the higher vibrations, the greater flow of energy. Begin using the Master symbol, familiarizing yourself with its power. Meditate on it. Practice attunements over a pillow or a teddy bear, until you feel confident that you can remember all the steps of the process. There's no hurry. You're going to be a Reiki Master for the rest of your life—which could be another 20, 40, or 60 years or more. You've got plenty of time to "grow up" in Reiki, because even when you've received a Master attunement, even if before that you've had many years of practice since Reiki 1, in Reiki terms you're still a baby! There's a lot of learning and growing to do before you become the equivalent of a Reiki teenager or young adult (in about 15 to 20 years' time), so there will be times of rebellion, times when you'll say to yourself, "Why on earth did I do this?" or "I'm sick of these rules, I'm going to do it my way." But of course there'll also be times of intense beauty and wonder, too, when you'll say, "I'm so glad I did this."

As in the case of the other Reiki courses, after being attuned as a Reiki Master you will go through another 21-day clearing cycle, but it does tend to be a bit deeper in its effects, as one might expect, since the Master energy has a very high vibration, so I would suggest that you don't attune anyone else for at least three months, and preferably six months or longer. Of course, you might choose not to attune anyone for many years, preferring to use the higher energies and the Master symbol for your own personal and spiritual development, and in your Reiki treatments on yourself and others, and that's fine. Let yourself go at a pace that suits you, and don't feel pressured by family or friends, who might be looking forward to you attuning them. Only do it when you feel it's right, and trust your inner instincts, your intuition, to let you know when that is.

BEING A REIKI MASTER

The role of Reiki Master is that of a respected teacher, someone who knows Reiki "inside out." By that I mean someone who lives with Reiki as an essential part of their daily lives, as well as someone who has plenty of knowledge and experience of using Reiki in different ways. However, please realize that no Reiki Master knows *everything* about Reiki. Reiki is itself a teacher, so the longer a

Master uses and teaches it, the further along the path *toward* mastery they go. And for each Master, that is a very personal journey, because each Master has a different starting point. Each of us has a unique set of life experiences, and it is inevitable that these will influence how, when and why we came to Reiki. And of course being a Master isn't just about knowing how to attune someone, or how to carry out a Reiki class. It's also about knowing how to lead someone toward their own personal and spiritual fulfillment—without judgment, without censure, but with love and compassion. That is passing on the essence of Reiki. And that's what you get better at as the years go by.

Some Masters have a thorough knowledge of other complementary therapies, some have been meditating and pursuing a spiritual path for many years, some have a psychic background, while for others Reiki is their first major step along their spiritual path. Reiki Masters come from all walks of life, including commerce and industry, the legal professions and the armed forces, the caring professions and agriculture, and from all age groups from their twenties, to their eighties or even nineties. This diversity means that there is bound to be a Reiki Master somewhere whose approach will appeal to you, and who will therefore be just the right person to guide you through your personal Reiki path. And then you will become the right person to guide others on their Reiki paths.

NOT THE RIGHT PATH FOR YOU?

It is also perfectly fine if you *don't* want to become a Reiki Master. It is neither necessary nor right for everyone, and many people get as much as they need from working with Reiki at Second Degree, or even First Degree. So wherever your Reiki journey takes you, I wish you as much joy and satisfaction and blessings as I have had—and even more. Love, light and Reiki blessings to you all.

RESOURCES

USEFUL CONTACT ADDRESSES AND WEBSITES

Penelope Quest

For information about Reiki courses and other workshops with Reiki Master Penelope Quest, and for details of all her books and CDs:

Websites: www.reiki-quest.co.uk and
www.penelopequest.com
E-mail: info@reiki-quest.co.uk

REIKI TEACHERS AND PRACTITIONERS IN THE UK

For details of other Reiki Masters and Practitioners, and useful information about Reiki and other forms of healing, you might like to try the following organizations and websites:

The UK Reiki Federation
Website: www.reikifed.co.uk
E-mail: enquiry@reikifed.co.uk

The Reiki Association
Website: www.reikiassociation.org.uk
E-mail: co-ordinator@reikiassociation.org.uk

The Reiki Council
Website: www.reikicouncil.org.uk
E-mail: info@reikicouncil.org.uk

The General Regulatory Council for Complementary Therapies (GRCCT)
Website: www.grcct.org
E-mail: admin@grcct.org

The Reiki Alliance-UK and Ireland
Website: www.reikialliance.org.uk
E-mail: mail@reikialliance.org.uk

Reiki Healers and Teachers Society (RHATS)
Website: www.reikihealersandteachers.net
E-mail: info@reikihealersandteachers.net

National Federation of Spiritual Healers (The Healing Trust)
Website: www.nfsh.org.uk or
www.thehealingtrust.org.uk

British Complementary Medicine Association (BCMA)
Website: www.bcma.co.uk
E-mail: chair@bcma.co.uk

Institute for Complementary Medicine (ICM)
Website: www.i-c-m.org.uk
E-mail: infor@i-c-m.org.uk

REIKI TEACHERS AND PRACTITIONERS IN THE U.S.A. AND CANADA

The Reiki Alliance – Worldwide
P.O. Box 41, Cataldo, ID 83810-1041
Website: www.reikialliance.com
E-mail: info@reikialliance.com

Usui Shiki Ryoho (The Office of the Grand Master – Phyllis Furumoto and Paul Mitchell)
Website: www.usuireiki-ogm.com

The International Center for Reiki Training
(William Lee Rand)
21421 Hilltop St. #28, Southfield, MI 48034-1023
Website: www.reiki.org
E-mail: center@reiki.org

International Association of Reiki Professionals
P.O. Box 481, Winchester, MA 01890
Website: www.iarp.org
E-mail: info@iarp.org

Southwestern Usui Reiki Ryoho Association
P.O. Box 5162, Lake Montezuma, AZ 86342-5162
Website: www.reiho.org
E-mail: adonea@msn.com

The Radiance Technique International Association, Inc. (TRTIA)
P.O. Box 40570, St. Petersburg, FL 33743-0570;
Website: www.trtia.org
E-mail: TRTIA@aol.com

Canadian Reiki Association
Box 54570, 7155 Kingsway, Burnaby, BC, V5E 4J6
Website: www.reiki.ca
E-mail: reiki@reiki.ca

Usui-Do (Traditional Japanese Reiki),
The Usui-Do Foundation, Toronto, Ontario, Canada
Website: www.usui-do.org
E-mail: askme@usui-do.org

WORLDWIDE CONTACTS

Reiki Dharma (Frank Arjava Petter) - Translations
available in English, Spanish and German
Website: www.reikidharma.com
E-mail: Arjava@ReikiDharma.com

Australian Reiki Connection
Website: www.australianreikiconnection.com.au

Reiki Australia,
Website: www.reikiaustralia.com.au

International House of Reiki (Frans and Bronwen Stiene)
Website: www.reiki.net.au
E-mail: info@reiki.net.au

Shibumi International Reiki Association
Website: www.shibumireiki.org

Reiki New Zealand Inc.
Website: www.reiki.org.nz
E-mail: info@reiki.org.nz

The Wellness Directory
Website: www.wellnessdirectory.co.nz

The Reiki Association of Southern Africa
Website: www.reikiassociation.co.za

Reiki Masters Association of South Africa
Website: www.reikihealing.co.za

World Reiki Association
Website: www.worldreikiassociation.org

International Holistic Therapies Directories
Website: www.internationalholistictherapiesdirectories.com

FURTHER READING

The following books are my recommendations from the many available on each subject. I have placed them under headings to make it easier to find the topics you want to pursue, but many of them cover several categories.

ABUNDANCE THEORY

Boyes, Carolyn, *Cosmic Ordering in 7 Easy Steps,* HarperCollins, 2006

Byrne, Rhonda, *The Secret,* Simon & Schuster, 2006

Cainer, Jonathan, *Cosmic Ordering,* HarperCollins, 2006

Carlson, Richard, *Don't Sweat the Small Stuff About Money,* Hodder & Stoughton, 1998

Dyer, Wayne W., *Manifest Your Destiny,* HarperCollins, 1998

Edwards, Gill, *Life Is a Gift,* Piatkus, 2007

Hicks, Esther and Jerry, *Ask and It Is Given,* Hay House, 2005

———, *Money and the Law of Attraction,* Hay House, 2008

Horan, Paula, *Abundance Through Reiki,* Lotus Light Publications, 1995

Mohr, Barbel, *The 21 Golden Rules for Cosmic Ordering,* Hay House, 2011

EMOTIONS AND EMOTIONAL FREEDOM TECHNIQUE (EFT)

Feinstein, David, PhD, Donna Eden, and Gary Craig, *The Healing Power of EFT & Energy Psychology,* Piatkus, 2006

Gallo, Fred P., and Harry Vincenzi, *Energy Tapping*, New Harbinger Publications, 2000

Goleman, Daniel, *Emotional Intelligence*, Bloomsbury, 1996

Hamilton, Dr. David R., *Why Kindness Is Good for You*, Hay House, 2011

Hicks, Esther and Jerry, *The Astonishing Power of Emotions*, Hay House, 2008

——, *Getting into the Vortex*, Hay House, 2010

Lynch, Paul and Valerie, *Emotional Healing in Minutes*, Thorsons, 2001

McKenna, Paul, *I Can Make You Happy*, Bantam Press, 2011

Pert, Candace B., *Molecules of Emotion*, Pocket Books, 1999

ENERGY, AURAS AND CHAKRAS

Brennan, Barbara Ann, *Hands of Light,* Bantam Books, 1990

Eden, Donna, with David Feinstein, PhD, *Energy Medicine*, Jeremy P. Tarcher, 2008

Emoto, Masaru, *The Hidden Messages in Water,* Beyond Words Publishing, 2004

Hunt, Valerie V., *Infinite Mind—Science of the Human Vibrations of Consciousness*, Malibu Publishing Co, 1996

Judith, Anodea, *Wheels of Life*, Llewellyn Publications, 1999

Lipton, Bruce, *The Biology of Belief*, Hay House, 2011

McTaggart, Lynne, *The Field: The Quest for the Secret Force of the Universe*, Element, 2003

Simpson, Liz, *The Book of Chakra Healing*, Gaia Books Ltd, 2005

FENG SHUI

Kingston, Karen, *Clear Your Clutter with Feng Shui*, Piatkus, 2008
——, *Creating Sacred Space with Feng Shui*, Piatkus, 1996
Spear, William, *Feng Shui Made Easy*, North Atlantic Books, 2010
Too, Lillian, *The Fundamentals of Feng Shui*, Element, 1999

HEALING

Angelo, Jack, *Your Healing Power*, Piatkus, 1998
Bays, Brandon, *The Journey*, Harper Element, 2012
Chopra, Deepak, MD, *Quantum Healing*, Bantam Books, 1990
Edwards, Gill, *Conscious Medicine*, Piatkus, 2010
Gawain, Shakti, *The Four Levels of Healing*, Eden Grove Editions, 1997
Gerber, Richard, MD, *Vibrational Medicine for the 21st Century*, Piatkus, 2000
Lloyd, Alexander, and Ben Johnson, *The Healing Code*, Hodder & Stoughton, 2011
Myss, Caroline, PhD, *Why People Don't Heal and How They Can*, Bantam Books, 1998
Siegel, Bernie S., MD, *Love, Medicine & Miracles*, Rider, 1999

METAPHYSICAL CAUSES OF DISEASE

Dethlefsen, Thorwald, and Ruediger Dahlke, MD, *The Healing Power of Illness*, Vega Books, 2002
Hay, Louise L., *Heal Your Body*, Hay House, 2004
——, *You Can Heal Your Life*, Hay House, 2004
Shapiro, Debbie, *Your Body Speaks Your Mind*, Piatkus, 2007
——, *Healing Mind, Healing Body*, Collins & Brown, 2007

METAPHYSICAL LIVING

Edwards, Gill, *Living Magically*, Piatkus, 2009
——, *Stepping into the Magic*, Piatkus, 2010
Gawain, Shakti, *Living in the Light*, New World Library, 2012
Holden, Robert, *Shift Happens*, Hay House, 2011
Jeffers, Susan, *End the Struggle and Dance with Life*, Hodder
    Paperbacks, 2005
——, *Feel the Fear and Do It Anyway*, Vermilion, 2007
Millman, Dan, *The Life You Were Born to Live*, H. J. Kramer, 1992
——, *No Ordinary Moments*, H. J. Kramer, 1993
Scovel–Shinn, Florence, *The Game of Life and How to Play It*,
    Vermilion, 2005

NEURO-LINGUISTIC PROGRAMMING (NLP) AND TRANSACTIONAL ANALYSIS (TA)

Bandler, Richard, *Get the Life You Want*, Harper Element, 2008
——, *Make Your Life Great*, Harper Element, 2010
Dilts, Robert, Tim Hallbom, and Suzi Smith, *Beliefs—Pathways
    to Health and Well-Being*, Metamorphous Press, 1990
Mallows, Michael, and Joseph Sinclair, *Peace of Mind Is a Piece
    of Cake*, Crown House Publishing, 1998
McDermott, Ian, and Joseph O'Connor, *NLP and Health*,
    Thorsons, 2001
Steiner, Claudia M., *Scripts People Live*, Avalon Travel
    Publishing, 1990
Stewart, Ian, and Vann Joines, *TA Today*, Life Space Publishing,
    1987

PHYSICAL BODY AND NUTRITION

Atkinson, Dr. Mark, *The Mind Body Bible*, Piatkus, 2007

Batmanghelidj, F., MD, *Your Body's Many Cries for Water*, The Therapist Ltd, 1997

Bloom, William, *The Endorphin Effect*, Piatkus, 2001

Hartrig, Kirsten, and Dr. Nic Rowley, *You Are What You Eat*, Piatkus, 1997

Holford, Patrick, *New Optimum Nutrition Bible*, Piatkus 2004

———, *6 Weeks to Super Health*, Piatkus, 2002

———, *The 10 Secrets of 100% Healthy People*, Piatkus 2010

Roizen, Michael F., MD, and Mehmet C. Oz, MD, *You: The Owner's Manual*, Piatkus, 2005

Waugh, Anne, and Allison Grant, *Ross and Wilson Anatomy and Physiology in Health and Illness*, Churchill Livingstone, 2006

REIKI

Ellis, Richard, *Reiki and the Seven Chakras*, Vermilion, 2002

Hall, Mari, *Reiki for Common Ailments*, Piatkus, 1999

Lubeck, Walter, and Frank Arjava Petter, *Reiki Best Practices*, Lotus Press, 2003

Lubeck, Walter, Frank Arjava Petter, and William Lee Rand, *The Spirit of Reiki*, Pilgrims Publishing, 2004

Petter, Frank Arjava, *The Original Reiki Handbook of Dr. Mikao Usui*, Lotus Press, 1999

Quest, Penelope, *Living the Reiki Way*, Piatkus, 2010

———, *Reiki for Life*, Jeremy P. Tarcher/Penguin, 2010

———, *Self-Healing with Reiki*, Jeremy P. Tarcher/Penguin, 2012

Quest, Penelope, and Kathy Roberts, *The Reiki Manual*, Jeremy P. Tarcher/Penguin, 2011

Steine, Bronwen and Frans, *The Japanese Art of Reiki*, O Books, 2005

———, *The Reiki Sourcebook*, O Books, 2003

SPIRITUAL GROWTH

Armstrong, Karen, *Twelve Steps to a Compassionate Life*, The
 Bodley Head, 2011
Chopra, Deepak, *Reinventing the Body, Resurrecting the Soul*,
 Crown Publishing, 2009
Hicks, Esther and Jerry, *Ask and It Is Given*, Hay House, 2005
——, *Getting into the Vortex*, Hay House, 2010
Myss, Caroline, *Anatomy of the Spirit, Bantam Books*, 1997
——, *Sacred Contracts*, Bantam Books, 2002
Ruiz, Don Miguel, *The Four Agreements*, Amber-Allen
 Publishing, Inc., 1997
Tolle, Eckhart, *A New Earth: Awakening to Your Life's Purpose*,
 Penguin Books Ltd, 2006
——, *The Power of Now: A Guide to Spiritual Enlightenment*,
 Hodder Mobius, 2001
Walsch, Neale Donald, *Communion with God*, Hodder &
 Stoughton, 2000
——, *Conversations with God*, Books 1, 2 and 3, Hodder &
 Stoughton, 1996, 1997, 1998
——, *Friendship with God*, Hodder & Stoughton, 1999
——, *The New Revelations*, Hodder & Stoughton, 2003
——, *Tomorrow's God*, Hodder & Stoughton, 2004

THE POWER OF THOUGHT

Carnegie, Dale, *How to Stop Worrying and Start Living*, Pocket
 Books, 2004
Dyer, Wayne W., *Change Your Thoughts, Change Your Life*, Hay
 House, 2007
——, *You'll See It When You Believe It*, Arrow, 1990
Hicks, Esther and Jerry, *The Amazing Power of Deliberate Intent*,
 Hay House, 2006

Hamilton, David R., PhD, *The Contagious Power of Thinking*, Hay House, 2011

——, *How Your Mind Can Heal Your Body*, Hay House, 2008

——, *It's the Thought That Counts*, Hay House, 2005

Leahy, Dr. Robert L., *The Worry Cure*, Piatkus, 2006

VISUALIZATION AND GUIDED MEDITATION

For CDs from Penelope Quest—
  Website: www.reiki-quest.co.uk
  E-mail: info@reiki-quest.co.uk

For tapes/CDs from Gill Edwards—
  Website: www.livingmagically.co.uk
  E-mail: info@livingmagically.co.uk

For CDs from William Bloom—
  Website: www.williambloom.com

For CDs from Esther and Jerry Hicks—
  Website: www.abraham-hicks.com

INDEX

Note: page numbers in **bold** refer to diagrams; page numbers in *italics* refer to information contained in tables.